Intimacy

Intimacy: Clinical, Cultural, Digital and Developmental Perspectives applies a contemporary, psychoanalytic lens to the many facets of intimacy between people, from romantic and sexual relationships, to friendliness, as well as the ways intimacy is mediated by new digital technologies.

Identifying commonalities and differences between a range of approaches, including classical Freudian, attachment theory and interpersonal theory, the book includes case studies that highlight how intimacy is framed in a variety of relationships. It examines the line between privacy and intimacy, as well as how intimacy changes at different stages of one's lifespan.

From the friends we have to the pets we own, or the faith we follow, a cross-cultural perspective ensures that intimacy is conceived of as a broad, essential element underlying all human relationships. The intimacy between analyst and analysand is also examined.

This far-reaching book will interest both practicing and training psychoanalysts and psychotherapists, as well as those in related disciplines.

Gurmeet Kanwal, M.D., is Clinical Associate Professor of Psychiatry, Weill Medical College of Cornell University, and Supervising Psychoanalyst and Teaching Faculty, William Alanson White Institute of Psychiatry, Psychoanalysis & Psychology. He is co-editor (with Salman Akhtar) of *Bereavement: Personal Experiences and Clinical Applications* (Karnac, 2017). He practices in New York City.

Salman Akhtar, M.D., is Professor of Psychiatry at Jefferson Medical College and Training and Supervising Analyst at the Psychoanalytic Center of Philadelphia. He is the author/editor of over 90 books, including the most recent, *Mind, Culture, and Global Unrest* (Routledge, 2018).

"I don't believe that there exists another body of work that covers the broad subject of intimacy as thoroughly as this one. Intimacy, as well as privacy, is discussed, in particular, from a developmental framework and most uniquely, from a multicultural and multi-gendered framework. Included in this unique and most contemporary volume are pointed discussions of intimacy in the age of technology, intimacy in the therapeutic relationship, intimacy with lovers, intimacy with friends, intimacy with animals and intimacy with a supreme being. Any clinician is bound to benefit enormously from exposure to this edited book."

Irwin Hirsch, Ph.D., New York University Postdoctoral Program in Psychotherapy and Psychoanalysis; The William Alanson White Institute of Psychiatry, Psychoanalysis & Psychology

"Who amongst us does not want to know more about the topic of intimacy? And, this book provides all of us a great opportunity to do so. From Akhtar's masterful introduction through Kanwal's perspicacious chapter to Bohm's concluding commentary, the reader repeatedly encounters rich, sophisticated, and nuanced discussion of various facets of intimacy. These include intimacy in love, friendship, spirituality, man's relationship with animals, and, most importantly, intimacy in the clinical situation. This book is a delight both for the intellect and the emotions!"

Aisha Abbasi, M.D., Training and Supervising Analyst, Michigan Psychoanalytic Institute, Author of *Rupture of Serenity* (2014)

Intimacy

Clinical, Cultural, Digital and Developmental Perspectives

Gurmeet Kanwal and
Salman Akhtar

Routledge
Taylor & Francis Group
LONDON AND NEW YORK

First published 2019
by Routledge
2 Park Square, Milton Park, Abingdon, Oxon OX14 4RN

and by Routledge
52 Vanderbilt Avenue, New York, NY 10017

Routledge is an imprint of the Taylor & Francis Group, an informa business

Chapter 1 is reprinted, with the author's and the publisher's permission, from *Silent Virtues: Patience, Curiosity, Privacy, Intimacy, Humility, and Dignity*, pp. 86–112. London: Routledge, 2019.

British Library Cataloguing-in-Publication Data
A catalogue record for this book is available from the British Library

Library of Congress Cataloging-in-Publication Data
Names: Kanwal, Gurmeet (Psychologist), editor. | Akhtar, Salman, 1946 July 31– editor.
Title: Intimacy / [edited by] Gurmeet Kanwal and Salman Akhtar.
Description: New York : Routledge, 2019. | Includes bibliographical references and index.
Identifiers: LCCN 2018041127 (print) | LCCN 2018052711 (ebook) | ISBN 9780429023217 (Master eBook) | ISBN 9780367085926 (hardback) | ISBN 9780367085940 (pbk.)
Subjects: LCSH: Intimacy (Psychology) | Interpersonal relations.
Classification: LCC BF575.I5 (ebook) | LCC BF575.I5 .I58 2019 (print) | DDC 158.2—dc23
LC record available at https://lccn.loc.gov/2018041127

ISBN: 978-0-367-08592-6 (hbk)
ISBN: 978-0-367-08594-0 (pbk)
ISBN: 978-0-429-02321-7 (ebk)

Typeset in Times New Roman
by Apex CoVantage, LLC

To

Bari

G.S.K.

Muge

S.A.

Contents

Acknowledgments

Eight distinguished colleagues devoted much time and effort to writing original works for inclusion in this book. They responded to our editorial suggestions with the utmost grace and patience. Oliver Rathbone, Rod Tweedy and Cecily Blench at Karnac Books shepherded this project through various stages of publication. Kate Pearce provided excellent and patient editorial assistance. My (S.A.) assistant, Jan Wright, prepared the manuscript of this book with her characteristic diligence and good humor. To all the individuals mentioned here, our sincere thanks indeed.

About the editors and contributors

Salman Akhtar, M.D., is Professor of Psychiatry at Jefferson Medical College and a Training and Supervising Analyst at the Psychoanalytic Center of Philadelphia. He has served on the editorial boards of the *International Journal of Psychoanalysis*, the *Journal of the American Psychoanalytic Association* and the *Psychoanalytic Quarterly*. His more than 300 publications include 82 books, of which the following 18 are solo-authored: *Broken Structures* (1992), *Quest for Answers* (1995), *Inner Torment* (1999), *Immigration and Identity* (1999), *New Clinical Realms* (2003), *Objects of Our Desire* (2005), *Regarding Others* (2007), *Turning Points in Dynamic Psychotherapy* (2009), *The Damaged Core* (2009), *Comprehensive Dictionary of Psychoanalysis* (2009), *Immigration and Acculturation* (2011), *Matters of Life and Death* (2011), *The Book of Emotions* (2012), *Psychoanalytic Listening* (2013), *Good Stuff* (2013), *Sources of Suffering* (2014), *No Holds Barred* (2016) and *A Web of Sorrow* (2017). Dr. Akhtar has delivered many prestigious invited lectures including a Plenary Address at the 2nd International Congress of the International Society for the Study of Personality Disorders in Oslo, Norway (1991), an Invited Plenary Paper at the 2nd International Margaret S. Mahler Symposium in Cologne, Germany (1993), an Invited Plenary Paper at the Rencontre Franco-Americaine de Psychanalyse meeting in Paris, France (1994), a Keynote Address at the 43rd IPA Congress in Rio de Janiero, Brazil (2005), the Plenary Address at the 150th Freud Birthday Celebration sponsored by the Dutch Psychoanalytic Society and the Embassy of Austria in Leiden, Holland (2006), and the Inaugural Address at the first IPA-Asia Congress in Beijing, China (2010). Dr. Akhtar is the recipient of numerous awards including the American Psychoanalytic Association's Edith Sabshin Award (2000), Columbia University's Robert Liebert Award for Distinguished Contributions to Applied Psychoanalysis (2004), the American Psychiatric Association's Kun Po Soo Award (2004) and Irma Bland Award for being the Outstanding Teacher of Psychiatric Residents in the country (2005). He received the highly prestigious Sigourney Award (2012) for distinguished contributions to psychoanalysis. In 2013, he gave the Commencement Address at graduation ceremonies of the Smith College School of Social Work in Northampton, MA. Dr. Akhtar's books have been translated in many languages, including German, Italian, Korean, Romanian, Serbian, Spanish and Turkish. A true Renaissance man, Dr. Akhtar has served as the Film Review Editor for the *International Journal of Psychoanalysis* and is currently serving as the Book Review Editor for the *International Journal of Applied Psychoanalytic Studies*. He has published nine collections of poetry and serves as a Scholar-in-Residence at the Inter-Act Theatre Company in Philadelphia.

Suzanne Benser, M.D., is a faculty member of the Psychoanalytic Center of Philadelphia (PCOP) and the immediate Past Chair of its administrative board. She also holds faculty appointments and medical staff appointments at Temple University, Pennsylvania Hospital and Einstein Medical Center of Philadelphia, and a previous faculty appointment at University of Pennsylvania. She leads a joint research project with PCOP and a school for foster children that provides psychoanalytic psychotherapy for at-risk youth. Dr. Benser has served as a bi-lingual group leader for Spanish-speaking players at Major League Baseball's Rookie Career Development Program for five consecutive years. She is a member of the American Psychoanalytic Association, Division 39/IX Psychoanalysis for Social Responsibility and the Racism Study Group. She has published a book chapter on prejudice and has a particular interest in developing ideas that bridge intrapsychic, intersubjective and interpersonal theories. Dr. Benser maintains a private practice of psychotherapy and psychoanalysis in Bala Cynwyd, PA.

Lori C. Bohm, Ph.D., is a Fellow, Supervising Analyst and Faculty member at the William Alanson White Institute. She is past Director of the Center for Applied Psychoanalysis and the Intensive Psychoanalytic Psychotherapy Program, William Alanson White Institute. She is an Associate Editor for *Contemporary Psychoanalysis*. She has co-edited a number of books with Brent Willock and Rebecca Curtis, including *Psychoanalytic Perspectives on Passion, Loneliness and Longing*, and *Psychoanalytic Perspectives on Identity and Difference*. She maintains a private practice in New York City and Hastings on Hudson, New York.

Todd Essig, Ph.D., is a Training and Supervising Psychoanalyst at the William Alanson White Institute. He has served on the editorial boards for *Contemporary Psychoanalysis* and the *Journal of the American Psychoanalytic Association* and was guest co-editor (with Gillian Isaacs Russell) for *Psychoanalytic Perspectives'* special issue on technology. For 16 years, until 2009, he was Director and Founder of The Psychoanalytic Connection (psychoanalysis.net), becoming widely known among colleagues as a pioneer in the innovative uses of information technologies for psychotherapists and other mental health professionals. In the aftermath of 9/11 he helped organize and served as Board Chair for the New York Disaster Counseling Coalition (NYDCC). He currently writes "Managing Mental Wealth" for *Forbes* where he covers the intersection of technology, public life and private experience. His clinical practice is in New York City where he treats individuals and couples, almost all of whom come to his office.

April Fallon, Ph.D., is the Faculty Chair and Professor at Fielding Graduate University, and Clinical Professor in Psychiatry at Drexel College of Medicine. She received her baccalaureate degree from Allegheny College (1975) and a Doctor of Philosophy in Psychology at the University of Pennsylvania (1981). She has received numerous awards for her teaching of psychiatric medical residents including the Psychiatric Educator 2012 from Philadelphia Psychiatric Society. She has co-authored five books with Virginia Brabender: *Models of Inpatient Group Psychotherapy* (1993), *Awaiting the Therapist's Baby: A Guide for Expectant Parent-Practitioners* (2003), *Essentials of Group Therapy* (2004), *Group Development in Practice: Guidance for Clinicians and Researchers on Stages and Dynamics of Change* (2009) and *The Impact of Parenthood on the Therapeutic Relationship* (2018). She has also co-edited an additional volume, *Working with Adoptive Parents: Research, Theory and Therapeutic Interventions* (2013). In addition, she has researched and written on the development of disgust in children and adults, body image and eating disorders, the effects of childhood maltreatment, and attachment and adoption. Dr. Fallon maintains a private practice in Ardmore, PA.

Rama Rao Gogineni, M.D., is Head of the Division of Child Psychiatry at Cooper University Hospital and a Clinical Professor in Psychiatry at Cooper Medical School of Rowan University. He received his M.D. degree from Osmania University in India (1972). He completed his residency in General Psychiatry at the University of Pennsylvania (1979) and his Child and Adolescent fellowship at Medical College of Pennsylvania (1982). He also obtained a master's degree in Family Therapy from Family Institute of Philadelphia. He completed his psychoanalytic training with Psychoanalytic Center of Philadelphia. Dr. Gogineni has served as President of Philadelphia Psychiatric Society, Regional Council of Child and Adolescent Psychiatry of Eastern Pennsylvania and Southern New Jersey, South Asian American Forum, and American Association for Social Psychiatry. He is a Distinguished Fellow of the American Psychiatric Association, the Academy of Child & Adolescent Psychiatry, and a member of the American College of Psychiatrists. He has written and presented on various aspects of fatherhood including depression, longing, adoption and immigration. He maintains a private practice in Bala Cynwyd, PA.

Gurmeet Kanwal, M.D., is Clinical Associate Professor of Psychiatry at the Weill Medical College of Cornell University, New York, where he teaches and supervises residents at the Payne Whitney Psychiatric Clinic. He is Supervising Psychoanalyst and Teaching Faculty at the William Alanson White Institute of Psychiatry, Psychology and Psychoanalysis, and past President of the William Alanson White Psychoanalytic Society. He is on the editorial boards of the

International Journal of Psychoanalysis and *Psychoanalytic Discourse*. Dr. Kanwal has co-edited (with Salman Akhtar) the book *Bereavement: Personal Experiences and Clinical Applications* (Karnac Books, London, 2017). His recent papers have appeared in *Psychoanalytic Review*, *Neuro-psychoanalysis and Psychoanalysis, Culture & Society*. He has also blogged for the *Psychoanalysis 3.0/Psychology Today* website and lectured in New Delhi, India and Tehran, Iran on interpersonal psychoanalysis. His areas of interest include culture, trauma and the interface of neuroscience and psychoanalysis. He is in full time private practice in New York City.

Danielle Magaldi, Ph.D., is a practicing psychologist and Associate Professor at The City University of New York, Lehman College. Her published research focuses on two areas: spirituality and technology in psychotherapy. Her publications on spirituality center on mindfulness, spiritual self-disclosure and the challenges that arise as secular psychologists treat religious patients. Publications on technology explore how technology is impacting therapeutic communication and intimacy. She received the Distinguished New Faculty Award for research on multicultural issues in education and counseling, and she sits on the editorial board of *Journal of Special Education Apprenticeship*. She is currently a candidate at New York University's Postdoctoral Program in Psychotherapy and Psychoanalysis and maintains a clinical practice in New York City treating adolescents, adults and couples.

Siamak Movahedi, Ph.D., is Professor of Sociology at the University of Massachusetts, Boston. He is also Professor of Psychoanalysis, Training and Supervising Analyst, and the Director of The Institute and the Doctoral Program in the Study of Psychoanalysis, Society & Culture at the Boston Graduate School of Psychoanalysis, and is likewise Training and Supervising Analyst at the HamAva Institute of Psychotherapy, Tehran, Iran. Professor Movahedi is the North America Editor of *Psychoanalytic Discourse*. He is a member of the American Psychoanalytic Association, American Psychological Association and International Psychoanalytic Association. He is the author of numerous papers and chapters in books and major national and international journals in psychoanalysis, psychology and sociology that have appeared among others in *American Imago*, *American Psychologist*, *American Sociological Review*, *Contemporary Psychoanalysis*, *Journal of the American Psychoanalytical Association*, *Journal of Health and Social Behavior*, *Modern Psychoanalysis*, *Canadian Journal of Psychoanalysis*, *International Journal of Psychoanalysis*, *International Forum of Psychoanalysis*, *L'Année Psychanalytique Internationale*, *Internationale Psychoanalyse Band 9: Moderne Pathologien*, *L'Annata Psicoanal. Int.*, and *Psychoanalytic Review*. His recent book chapter, "The Narcissism of Minor Differences: The Status Anxiety & Disciplinary Intolerance between Sociology and Psychoanalysis", appeared in *The Unhappy Divorce of Sociology and Psychoanalysis* (2014). His recent papers include "Contextualized Language and Transferential Aspects of Context", *Journal of the American Psychoanalytic Association* (2015); "A False Dichotomy between Science and Hermeneutics, and Observation and Interpretation in the Analysis of Manifest Dreams in Clinical Work", *Psychoanalytic Discourse* (2017); and his two co-authored papers with Nahaleh Moshtagh, "Your Smartphone Is Watching You: Evocative Objects of Influence and Fear of Breakdown", *Psychoanalytic Review* (2016); and "Persian Tales on the Couch: Notes on Folktales as the Mirror of the Contemporary Cultural Struggles with Gender and Sexuality", *International Forum of Psychoanalysis* (2018).

David Pauley, L.C.S.W., is a Training and Supervising Psychoanalyst and member of the faculty at the Psychoanalytic Psychotherapy Study Center. He holds an M.A. in French Studies and an M.S.W. from New York University, and completed training in psychoanalytic psychotherapy and psychoanalysis, respectively, at PPSC and Mid-Manhattan Institute for Psychoanalysis. His recent paper, "The Negative Transitional Object: Theoretical Elaboration and Clinical Illustration", was published in a March 2018 issue of *Psychoanalytic Dialogues*. His clinical writing has also appeared in the *Journal of Gay and Lesbian Psychotherapy*, *Annals of Modern Psychoanalysis*, and the *Journal of College Student Psychotherapy*. He maintains a private practice in Brooklyn where he works with adults, teenagers, children, couples and groups.

Christie Platt, Ph.D., is a Psychoanalyst and Clinical Psychologist in Washington, DC. Her private practice encompasses a diverse population including university students, adult professionals and veterans of both the Iraq and Afghanistan wars. Dr. Platt's writings on intersubjectivity, issues of race and ethnicity, and the arts, have been published in various publications including the *American Journal of Psychoanalysis*. A Teaching Analyst at the Baltimore Washington Center for Psychoanalysis, she received her doctorate from the California School of Professional Psychology in Berkeley, CA. Dr. Platt is currently writing a memoir about the year she hitchhiked 9,000 miles on her way from Cape Town, South Africa to Cairo, Egypt.

Bari Smelson-Kanwal, L.C.S.W., Ph.D., is a Clinical Social Worker and Psychoanalyst, with extensive experience doing therapy with individuals, couples, families and groups. She is Teaching Faculty at the Westchester Center for the Study of Psychoanalysis and Psychotherapy, where she teaches and supervises in the couples therapy program. She is a past Adjunct Professor of Social Work at New York University and Mercy College. Her group therapy training was with the Eastern Group Psychotherapy Society. She has lectured in Delhi, India on couples therapy, combining systems theory and psychoanalysis. Her interests include the effect of an offspring's mental illness on the mother, and issues of race, ethnicity, faith and culture in multicultural couples. She has a private practice in New York City and Dobbs Ferry, NY.

Leora Trub, Ph.D., is an Associate Professor of Psychology at Pace University in the school/clinical-child Psy.D. program, where she is involved in clinical training, supervision and teaching of future psychologists. She founded the Digital Media and Psychology lab at Pace University, which examines the intersection between psychology and technology, with a focus on how technologies affect our conception of ourselves and our relationship with others, and what underlying psychological and emotional needs they meet. Among her projects are the development and testing of a mindfulness app aimed at increasing people's awareness of themselves and others during text-based interactions, and an in-depth examination of how technology alters the psychotherapy frame and impacts clinical practice. She is also in private practice in downtown Manhattan, where she works with adolescents, adults and couples.

to the experience of intimacy, according to Rubin. Mention of 'closeness' brings up Burch's (2004) interesting viewpoint which holds closeness and intimacy to lie on a continuum. He sees closeness as being in the conscious realm and intimacy as arising from the unconscious. Closeness does not preclude intimacy but does not necessarily include it. Physical proximity and frequency of contact can lead to 'closeness' but not necessarily to 'intimacy'.[2] Moreover, intense engagement with another person can exist without closeness, for instance, during states of anger (Schimel, 1987). Shared situations of fear (e.g. disasters) and excitement (e.g. football games) can lead to closeness with others without actual intimacy. Perhaps closeness refers to sharing focal areas of experience whereas intimacy involves much greater trust and a more diffuse and far-reaching psychological nakedness on the part of the two parties involved.

Putting such speculation aside, I return to Burch and note that he gives premium to the experience of 'tenderness' in the context of intimacy. He cites Thorne (1991) who declared that "when tenderness is present in a relationship, I believe there is the possibility of finding wholeness and of recognizing the liberating paradox" (p. 77); giving oneself over to someone leaves nothing to be desired anymore and taking someone in fully allows them to be truly themselves.[3] Though neither Thorne nor Burch mention it, the work of preeminent Finnish psychoanalyst, the late Veikko Tähkä (1993) is outstanding in this context. Tähkä described tenderness as an affect arising from

> empathic sharing of the object's pleasure and subsequent leaving of the pleasure for him. In a loving relationship, this letting the object keep the pleasure for himself is followed by a second re-pleasure in the subject for the loved person's feeling and for the knowledge of having contributed to that oneself. (p. 244)

The maternal quality of this experience brings up the issue of gender-transcendence during intimacy. Brody (1978) emphasizes that "true intimacy may require the abandonment of some conventional aspects of gender identity" (p. 521) giving credence to Binstock's (1973) earlier statement that "the state of being in love completes the lover's identity as part of a male-female duality" (p. 104). And, it is true that identification with the partner's excitement during sex makes it possible to derive pleasure from his or her erotic desire. Kernberg (1995) notes that under such circumstances, there is a sense of

> temporarily overcoming the ordinarily unbreachable barrier separating the genders, and a sense of completion and enjoyment of the penetrating and encompassing, penetrated and enclosed aspect of sexual invasion. In this connection the symbolic displacement of all "penetrating" parts of the anatomy and of all "penetrable" openings signals the condensation of eroticism from all zones . . . and the consequent confluence, in sexual activity or contact, of

> fantasies and experiences reflecting the entire body surface of both participants. . . . Unconsciously identifying with both genders eliminates the need to envy the other gender, and, in remaining oneself while becoming the other as well, one has a sense of having achieved intersubjective transcendence. (p. 23)

While marked during the actual sexual encounter, a loosening of roles customarily held proper for one or the other gender occurs in most states of intimacy within a romantic couple. This is more 'visible' among heterosexual couples but no less true for homosexual dyads, even though their intrapsychic traffic across genders is more layered and nuanced.

All in all, the experience of romantic intimacy involves the following seven characteristics: (i) physical and emotional closeness; (ii) trust in the essential goodness of the partner; (iii) relaxation of personal boundaries; (iv) overcoming of shame about one's actual or imaginary blemishes and gently overcoming the partner's proclivity to shame; (v) sharing of private thoughts, fantasies, emotions and expectations; (vi) empathic immersion in the subjectivity of the other; (vii) tenderness, i.e. joy in the other's self-realization and in facilitating that to occur; and (viii) oscillating and partial transcendence of gender boundaries. Intimacy in non-romantic contexts, such as friendship, follows the same pattern though the erotic element is not integral to it (or is 'aim-inhibited')[4] and there is lesser requirement for gender transcendence. While sex dissolves gender boundaries, friendships solidify them. This is true of both same gender and cross-gender friendships.

Developmental substrate

While Erikson's (1968) declaration that it is "only when identity formation is well on its way that true intimacy – which is really a counterpointing as well as fusing of identities – is possible" (p. 135) seems true, it is also true that the foundations of the capacity for intimacy are laid down in the earliest stages of infancy and childhood. The components of intimacy, especially those subsumed under the 'affectionate current' (Freud, 1910) of love, include trust, concern, porousness of self-boundaries, mutuality, absence of shame, sharing of experiences and tenderness. All of them have their origins in early mother-child relationship and to this we must turn at this point.

With differing metaphors and theoretical lexicon, all important theoreticians of early development emphasize that a comfortable fit between the infant and its mother is the basis of psychic stability, safety and confidence. Concepts such as 'absolute dependence' (Fairbairn, 1952), 'primary attachment bond' (Bowlby, 1969), the state of 'illusion' (Winnicott, 1960b) and 'dual-unity' (Mahler, Pine, & Bergman, 1975) all indicate that the availability of reliable maternal care leads the child to develop trust in its own abilities and to evolve a benevolent view of the world at large. Benedek's (1938) and Erikson's (1950) notions of 'confident expectation' and 'basic trust', respectively, speak to this very point.

With such self-assurance and a charitable world view, the growing child becomes capable of forays in external reality; continued access to the primary object for "emotional refuelling" (Furer, cited in Mahler et al., 1975, p. 69) helps sustain the necessary 'we-ness' (Bergman, 1980, 1999) during such assertions of 'me-hood'. By the time the child acquires self- and object-constancy, he can defer gratification, indulge in fantasy enactments and enjoy role-playing. Fusion of good and bad object representations enhances his capacity to cope with simultaneous love and anger towards self and others (Kernberg, 1975). By age 3 or so, the average child can attend nursery school, showing that he is capable to accept a mother substitute. His dialogue with his internalized mother makes it possible for him to feel a modicum of intimacy with his kindergarten teacher (Kramer, 1996). Still later, during the oedipal period, sexual curiosities arise and the nature of parental intimacy becomes a matter of great concern for the child. He tries to understand sexual matters and succeeds to a certain extent, but many things still remain mysterious. Repression then sets in, leading to compartmentalization of the mind, layering of the self and aim-inhibition of erotic desires typical of this developmental period (Freud, 1924).

During the subsequent phase of latency (from 6 to 12 years or so), relationship with school teachers and same-sex peers broadens the child's emotional arena. Friendships in latency and, later on, during adolescence allow sharing secret ambitions and sexual curiosities. Much intimacy characterizes such relationships as they are replete with exclusivity, mutuality and tenderness. The onset of adolescence especially pushes the young individual towards seeking intimacy, this time with a romantic and sexual partner. Love and sex, hitherto existing as separate, now come to be fused. Counterphobic disidentification with parents (Blos, 1967; Tyson & Tyson, 1990) and 'hyper-intimacy' with peers in the service of identity consolidation gradually settles and a return to conventionality becomes evident. This marks the beginning of young childhood. Parents are still loved and so are friends, but deeper confidences are now shared only with one's romantic partner (homosexual or heterosexual, with or without marriage). Becoming a parent oneself and raising children opens up new avenues for intimacy with one's partner. Still later, the accrual of shared memories offers the intimacy of mutual nostalgia. At the terminal end of life, accommodations to changes in biological functioning propel the couple to seek novel ways of sustaining romantic intimacy (Kaplan, 1990). Clearly, throughout the lifespan, psychological health

> includes the idea of tingling life and the magic of intimacy. All these things go together and add up to a sense of feeling real and of being, and of the experiences feeding back into the personal psychic reality, enriching it, and giving it scope. The consequence is that the healthy person's inner world is related to the outer or actual world and yet is personal and capable of an aliveness of its own . . . each person has a polite or socialized self, and also a personal private self that is not available except in intimacy.
>
> (Winnicott, 1984, pp. 31, 66)

To this relatively 'conservative' survey of developmental literature, one must add some significant newer contributions. The following six certainly merit inclusion here though much more literature than I can cover exists in this realm. I summarize them in chronological order of their appearance.

Levenson (1984) proposed that the mother's differing attitudes towards her male and female offspring contribute to the differences between their varying patterns of closeness and distance from her: "While the boy can differentiate via gender, the girl must struggle to differentiate via generation" (p. 531). Boundaries remain more porous for the latter as she grows further. As a result "at the point of marriage – the adult intimate dyad – a man's basic issue is how to be intimate and *stay* autonomous; a woman's is still how to be intimate and *become* autonomous" (p. 533, italics in the original).

Horner (1986) devoted a monograph to the tension between the search for intimacy and the desire to preserve independence and authenticity. She traced the healthy capacity to strike a balance between these polarities back to the amalgamation of the mother's supportive-holding activities on the one hand and individuation-promoting functions on the other.

Stern (1985), in his well-received book, *The Interpersonal World of the Infant*, highlighted the interactional synchrony between the mother and her baby *and* the mother's joy in the child's pleasure in his efficacy as the founding units of mutuality and intimacy in the child. Stern described four stages of developing self: emergent, core, subjective and verbal. It is only at the third stage (beginning around 8 months of age) that actual intersubjective exchange with mother becomes possible. Capacity for intimacy is born at this point. Revisiting his book 13 years later, Stern (1998) added the concept of 'narrative self' which followed the 'verbal self'. This constellation gives rise to the first true and false stories one develops about oneself; these can include facts and fictions about one's capacity or incapacity for intimacy with others.

Ehrlich (1998) delineated two experiential modalities, those of 'being' and 'doing'. Both must be present for consolidation of identity and healthy functioning of the self. Ehrlich went on to say that:

> A resolution of intimacy based exclusively on the modality of *Doing* will at best be a portrait of drive domination and will never extend far beyond the erotic question of who is doing what to whom. On the other hand, intimacy that is resolved exclusively in the *Being* modality will be of the kind encountered in deep spiritual unions, like those met in intensive religious and mystical experiences. Exclusively, unalloyed to at least a modicum of what can be provided by the *Doing* modality, it cannot provide an alternative to the necessary encounter between members of opposite genders, whose mental, spiritual, physical, and instinctual union leads to cross-fertilization, offspring, and family formation.
>
> (p. 157, italics in the original)

Alperin (2001) emphasized that the need for intimacy is inborn and finds strength from empathic attunement between the infant and its mother. The adult desire for intimacy reflects a wish to return to this early stage and "undo the primordial separation from the mother" (p. 140). Alperin included the following among obstacles to intimacy in adulthood: the 'alienating individualism' (Rotenberg, 1977) of capitalist societies, fear of psychic dissolution during closeness, paranoid hostility and incestuous anxieties.

Orbach (2007) focused upon this last issue and explored it in the context of romantic couples. She noted that in such a setting, three different attachment schemas are at work: that of each individual and that of the entity itself. This last one is what matters in the end. Helping to elevate it above individual attachment patterns and safeguarding the space it provides in the form of 'separated attachment' and 'connected autonomy' makes it possible for the couple to recover and/or sustain sexual intimacy between them.

Finally, I wish to add a developmental notion of my own. This pertains to there being some difference between the sort of intimacy a child has with its mother and with its father. 'Maternal intimacy' is overarching, not necessarily verbal, and provides psychic nourishment and sustenance. 'Paternal intimacy' is focal, didactic and geared toward external reality.[5] Superimposed on top of these are the different types of intimacies with the same-sex and the opposite-sex parent. In the girl's case, the 'maternal intimacy' and the 'same-sex parent intimacy' are harmonious; this deepens the capacity for intimacy in her but also increases the fear of autonomy. In the boy's case, the 'maternal intimacy' and the 'same-sex parent intimacy' involve two different figures; this weakens the capacity for intimacy but increases the regressive fear of merger. I will return to how these two forms of relatedness act in unison in the technical section of this paper. Before discussing such technical issues, however, it is necessary to consider scenarios where things have gone wrong and where the possibility of intimacy is grossly compromised.

Psychopathology

Like all character traits, capacity for intimacy is subject to derailments of personality development, psychic trauma and unfortunate vicissitudes of adult life. Morbid forms of intimacy thus emerge. These include: (i) failed intimacy, (ii) florid intimacy, (iii) fluctuating intimacy and (iv) false intimacy. Brief comments on each follow.

Failed intimacy

Not all people are capable of developing and sustaining intimate relationships with others. Their efforts to achieve intimacy fail due to various deficit and defense-based impediments from within. Four levels of psychopathology are generally evident under such circumstances. The *first level* pertains to schizoid anxieties regarding emotional closeness with another person. As a child, the schizoid has felt chronically unloved and unseen in his psychic veracity by his parents (Ferenczi, 1929; Fairbairn, 1952). His overtures of playfulness and love were treated as intrusions by them. As an adult, he dreads expressing his affectionate and needy feelings to others lest these be rejected all over again. He relates to them via intellect and reason, becoming didactic or preachy in the process. Others do not understand him, cannot relate to his aloofness and, at times, feel intimidated by him. Consequently, the schizoid individual finds himself devoid of friendships. There is little or no genuine intimacy in his life since he dreads (and, using rationalization, derides) the ordinary messiness and unpredictability of human relationships.

The *second level* of failed intimacy is caused by paranoid fears. After all, emotional closeness with others requires that one trusts the other person and finds it safe to be with him or her in a relaxed, self-disclosing way. This is difficult for individuals whose lives are structured around viewing themselves as the object of others' hostility, interference and oppression. They are suspicious and feel unjustly treated by others. As a result, they erect defensive walls of humorless rigidity and vigilance. As a character trait, mistrust becomes a formidable barrier to intimacy in both social and romantic spheres of life (see Akhtar, 2016, for details).

The *third level* of deficient empathy involves narcissistic character traits. Freud's (1914) 'U-tube theory' of the relationship between self-love and object-love still holds water: the more one loves oneself, the less one can love others. However, more nuances have come to be recognized in this context (Kohut, 1971, 1977; Kernberg, 1975, 1984; Akhtar, 1992a, 2009a; Bach, 1977). It has been noted that the narcissistic individual is forever busy burnishing the image he presents to others and this preoccupation siphons off the psychic energy needed to listen to others. He cannot grasp the psychic depth of others. And, if he presents himself as shining, perfect and above any criticism, then others cannot reach his inner self. Either way, the door to intimacy gets closed. Moreover, letting others know oneself requires acceptance of one's total self and not of one's strengths only. In other words, deep and genuine interaction with others requires humility[6] and the narcissist is incapable of self-effacement. To complicate matters further, knowing others fully has the dual risk of encountering their blemishes as well as their strengths. The former warrants restraint of criticism and the latter requires tolerance of envy. Both tasks are difficult for the narcissist and therefore he avoids intimacy with others. Yet another difficulty arises from the narcissist's profound internal attachment to "an ideal object with whom one would never have to feel aggression and from whom no aggressive actions would have to be tolerated" (Richards & Spira, 2003, p. 357). This condemns him to a never-ending search or life-long wait for this perfect object. Meanwhile, the capacity for meaningfully relating to imperfect and 'ordinary' objects is seriously compromised.

Finally, the *fourth level* of difficulty in achieving intimacy exists in the context of a neurotic or 'higher level of character organization' (Kernberg, 1970). Problems of this sort are generally milder in intensity, often ego-dystonic and limited in their relational scope. They mostly involve the sexual realm and manifest as inhibitions of pre-genital sexuality, especially during foreplay. Capable of trusting, deep and sustained bonds on a selective basis, individuals with neurotic restrictions of intimacy can end up with restricted sexuality and an unexciting social life suffused with 'unmentalized xenophobia' (Akhtar, 2007).

Regardless of the levels of psychopathology outlined above, a common defense against intimacy is to 'elevate' its lack into a proud insistence upon freedom.

> One experiences not the threat of intimacy, but that one needs space, can't stand coercion, loves freedom, isn't ready yet, and so forth. In its easiest formulation, the quest is for freedom and the avoidance of anything that compromises it. Commitment, even the idea of commitment, threatens that quest. To maintain freedom, affects and associations arising in opposition are censored within, through psychic defences. Hence, freedom-seeking persons, in extreme instances, need to avoid wishing for anything or caring about anyone. Intimacy with another and caring for another mobilize anxiety that is attenuated through denial, detachment, contempt, rationalization, and the sabotage of trust.
>
> (Ingram, 1986, p. 77)

In contrast to this spectrum of psychopathology leading to deficient or failed intimacy are situations and characters which facilitate the development of 'hyper-intimacy'.

Florid intimacy

Using the designation 'florid' in its sense of being extravagant and declamatory, I wish to describe characters and situations where a certain kind of ready-made bonhomie prevails and where intimacy develops quite rapidly between strangers or near-strangers. Five scenarios come to mind.

- Someone older, affluent and resourceful but deeply traumatized encounters a younger and financially compromised person with a similar traumatic background. The former has an uncanny empathy for the latter; he wants to 'rescue' the less fortunate of the duo. They develop a quick and tight bond of intimacy.
- A lonely immigrant poet living in a land where hardly anyone understands his language finds out that another poet of his language is visiting town. They meet. A long and intimate discourse ensues. In what Kretschmer (1925) called an "enlarged autism along people of similar persuasion" (p. 162), the two become deep friends and continue to communicate with each other long after the visiting poet returns to his land.
- In the living room of a Bollywood movie star, young aspirants spill their guts and on the slightest cue from the matinee idol reveal their deepest secrets. The star is not moved towards reciprocal disclosure but a fellow

'minor artist' present there (an 'extra' in old terminology of the film industry) becomes enamored and shares his or her private thoughts with fervent desire for closeness.
- A sexually perverse man and woman with mutual consent and with precisely matching depth of regression decide to eat each other's feces. They regard this ego-polluting ecstasy as evidence of their profound intimacy with each other.
- In contrast to this grotesque illustration is the following elegant passage describing the instantaneous development of intimacy between two sadomasochistic strangers. "The large wide-open eyes contain a hint of reproach. The gaze sinks deeply into me. She plays a fallen woman, the victim of a need for love that leads her repeatedly to villainous men who will use her and forsake her. She is stuck with her vulnerability, her hidden masochism, and I am stuck with my secret sadism. Across that gulf our glances meet, we recognize each other. We are a pair" (Wheelis, 1994, p. 86).

What all these illustrations have in common is the triad of (i) extraordinary porousness of self-boundaries, (ii) uncanny mutuality of 'tongues' between the parties involved and (iii) rapidity with which emotional engagement takes place between them. Situational (e.g. immigration, Bollywood drama), aesthetic (e.g. poetry, other common interests) and characterological variables (e.g. perversion, hypomanic tendencies) all contribute to the development of 'florid intimacy'. Let me hasten to add that rapid development of intimacy must not be reflexively devalued. To be sure, not all such instances have happy endings[7] and many evaporate with the speed with which they developed. However, some of them can give rise to long-term friendships. I fondly myself recall my first ever conversation with the London-based South African psychoanalyst Julian Stern, which lasted for 11 hours and has resulted in a deep and mutually gratifying and ongoing friendship of 25 years.

Fluctuating intimacy

Seemingly a coexistence of 'failed' and 'florid' intimacies, the syndrome of 'fluctuating intimacy' usually arises from an equipotent mixture of object hunger and merger anxieties (Guntrip, 1969; Mahler et al., 1975). Object hunger propels closeness and giving 'hundred percent' of oneself to others in the hope of becoming indispensable to them. Merger anxieties stir up fear of losing all autonomy and becoming enslaved. One's own object hunger is projected upon the object leading to fantasies of being cannibalized. As a result, such individuals (often termed 'borderline') withdraw from closeness. But this exposes them to the pain of stark aloneness and lack of belonging. Wanting to avoid this latter dread, they return to the object only to get anxious all over again. Like Schopenhauer's (1851) porcupines, partners caught in such a relational matrix fluctuate between intimacy and distance, trust and mistrust, betrayal and confession, and separateness and merger.

They cannot live peacefully together nor can they do without each other. For such individuals, emotional involvement stirs up a characteristic 'need-fear dilemma' (Burnham, Gladstone, & Gibson, 1969): to be intimate is to court engulfment and to be apart is to court aloneness. Not surprisingly, they keep going back and forth and remain inconsolable at either end of the intimacy-separateness spectrum (Gunderson, 1985; Melges & Swartz, 1989; Akhtar, 1990). That such oscillations of 'optimal distance' (Akhtar, 1992b) disrupt their relationships is beyond question. What remains dubious is whether their closeness with loved ones can be accorded the status of genuine intimacy. Their inability to accept others fully, metabolize aggression and master merger fears attendant upon close contact impede their grasp of others' subjectivity. Their 'intimacy' is not only transitory but superficial as well.

False intimacy

Since intimacy, by definition, means psychological integrity, interactional transparency, emotional truthfulness and mutual trust, any departure from these components contaminates the experience. Individuals who have not achieved self- and object-constancy (Mahler et al., 1975) and who lack the capacity for relating to 'whole objects' (Klein, 1935) can only muster pale facsimiles of intimacy; they relate from parts of their selves to parts of others.

Such developmentally determined failure is, however, not the main origin of false intimacy. Mandatory insertion of a part object or a lubricated accouterment of desire into romantic intimacy is what renders it false. Freud's (1927e) description of fetishism whereby an interposition of an inanimate object (e.g. shoe, earrings, stocking) or some part of the body (e.g. foot, lock of hair) becomes a requirement for a man's achieving sexual union with a woman is the prototype of false intimacy. Khan (1979) extended this theme and declared that "the pervert puts an *impersonal object* between his desire and his accomplice; this object can be a stereotyped fantasy, a gadget, or a pornographic image. All three alienate the pervert from himself, as, alas, from the object of his desire" (p. 9, italics in the original). Going into further details of the pervert's "technique of intimacy" (p. 20), Khan noted that such a person is incapable of relating to a truly separate object. For him, the object occupies an intermediary position: not entirely subjective and yet treated as subjectively created. Through such maneuver of intimacy, he "tries to *make known* to himself and *announce and press into* another something pertaining to his innermost nature as well as to discharge instinctual tension in a compulsive and exigent way" (p. 22, italics in the original). The relational consequences and the paradoxical pallor of such turgid closeness elicit the following eloquent passage from Khan.

> The capacity to create the emotional climate in which another person volunteers to participate is one of the few real talents of the pervert. This invitation to surrender to the pervert's logic of body-intimacies demands of the object

> a suspension of discrimination and resistance at all levels of guilt, shame, and separateness. A make-believe situation is offered in which two individuals temporarily renounce their separate identities and boundaries and attempt to create a heightened maximal body-intimacy of orgastic nature. There is always, however, one proviso. The pervert himself cannot surrender to the experience and retains a split-off, dissociated manipulative ego-control of the situation. This is both his achievement and failure in the *intimate* situation.
>
> (p. 22, italics in the original)

A more recent rendering of such pseudo-intimacy can be found in Celenza's (2015) clarification that in both male and female sexual perversions, the prevailing dynamics involve objectification of the woman's body. Pleasurable and orgastic though the interaction might be, it can hardly claim the status of being intimate since both partners have colluded in eliminating the subjectivity of the female partner, replacing it with complicity and dehumanizing compliance.

Outside of the sexual scenario, postures of false intimacy can also be discerned in the social lives of narcissistic and sociopathic characters (Kernberg, 1984, 1992; Akhtar, 1989, 1992a, 2007). Elsewhere, I have commented upon the former's inability in the following manner.

> He or she does not wish to renounce total autonomy while also not permitting a separate mental life to the other. Under the pressure of instinctual drives, the narcissistic individual comes too close to the other person and defending against the aggression, inevitably mobilized by intimacy, he withdraws and becomes cold and aloof. In contrast to the mature relatedness in love which gradually deepens, narcissistic relatedness is characterized by cycles of need-based intimacy and defensive withdrawals. Or, there develops a pattern of intense idealization and coercive control of the other with no deepening of actual knowledge of that person over time.
>
> (Akhtar, 2009a, pp. 102–103)

In the sociopathic character, corrosion of superego functions and deterioration of ethical foundations of human relatedness leads either to the total incapacity of intimacy or to a peculiar kind of transitory and false intimacy arising mostly out of "glibness and charm" (Abraham, 1925, p. 299) which pulls the other person close, and 'state-related empathy' (Gediman, 1985) which permits a sharp though transitory attunement to the other person's needs. The sociopath, like a skillful puppeteer, is able to seduce the other person to take steps towards intimacy while waiting to make his exploitative move.

Sociocultural aspects

Since intimacy, by definition, involves the relationship between two or more individuals, it is likely to be affected by a given society's provision of prototypes of such experience during childhood, facilitation of close interpersonal relationships during adult life and the endemic sustenance of belief in the value of human relatedness and mutuality. To be sure, all societies offer such avenues to its members. However, to the extent they do so differs. And, this difference can account for cross-cultural variations in the degree of intimacy and the value accorded to the experience.

In the age of the 'Protean Man' (Lifton, 1971) and the 'culture of narcissism' (Lasch, 1979), great emphasis is placed upon appearances, acquisitions, ambitions and self-benefitting 'adjustments' to circumstances. Family life suffers when parents are consumed by demands of work and pressure to make money. Childhood is aborted.[8] Children have fewer siblings and limited contact with their cousins, who often do not live in the same city. Miller (2013) eloquently describes the toll all this takes upon the emotional lives of children and I quote him at some length.

> The lot of children seems to have deteriorated in a number of ways. First and foremost, the combination of accelerating family breakdown and economic pressures requiring two incomes has meant that children have less and less personal relationship with their parents and virtually no experience of normal family life. Second, the dangers of road traffic and fear of paedophiles and other predators make it extremely rare for children to be able to play with their neighbors and friends unsupervised, and close to their home. The result is something of a siege mentality. Inside the "safe houses" (home, nursery school, school, after-school clubs, etc.) life is barren, two-dimensional, and stressful. During leisure hours, three-dimensional, practical experience of building, inventing, and constructing is a thing of the past. Computer graphics replace reality and the television screen and the headphone enforce passivity. School hours are dominated by the pressure of tests, attainment levels, examinations, inspections, and the coercive nature of league tables. The joy of learning and the importance of living co-operatively are replaced by the pressure to succeed and the preoccupation with competition.
>
> (pp. 200–201)

On an earlier, developmental level too, the contemporary scenario in the West (especially in the United States) seems grim. Capitalism thrives on the induction of 'false needs' (Akhtar, 2011) which makes people conclude that they have to make more money to purchase more things; this partly contributes to the unquestioned norm of the two-income family. Since paid maternity leave is short (e.g. six weeks in the U.S.A.), babies are put in 'day care', and then into 'preschool' centers. Mother-child bonding suffers and what is lost due to the lack of comfortable leaning upon the mother for care and assurance is 'compensated' by the familial and societal exaltation of autonomy. Expressions such as 'take care of yourself' and 'do it yourself' go unquestioned and 'assisted living', which is actually an existential requirement of all human beings, becomes a subtly derided accommodation for the elderly and terminally ill. The pallor of 'we-ness' produces a 'me-generation' that is replete with ambition, hesitant about dependency and compromised in the capacity for intimacy. Work-mates, especially in white-collar settings, do not socialize with each other. Friends know little about each other's personal problems and have to make appointments to share a meal often weeks and months in advance.

Matters are different in most Latin American, Mediterranean and Asian cultures. Though the juggernaut of American-style consumerism is beginning to impact these societies, their distinction from the North American norms is still noticeable. In many such places, women do not work outside the home, quit their jobs upon having babies or are afforded fully paid long maternity leave. Joint or extended families still exist and the child is not left with paid strangers from 6 weeks onwards (as is frequently the case in the United States). Often a group of women (mother, grandmother, aunts, older female siblings and cousins) are available to care for the child (Roland, 1988; Kurtz, 1992) and assure a certain continuity of skin-to-skin contact and emotional dependence. Children have more siblings and greater access to their maternal and paternal cousins. They play with each other and thus engage in the emotional lives of their peers on a regular basis. Neighbors constitute an important part of a relationship network. Ordinary human competitiveness is sacrificed at the altar of mutual respect and social cohesion. Workplace offers opportunities for life-long bonds. Friendships are deep and involve great sharing of information, personal feelings and even secrets. Intimacy abounds, and loneliness is exceptional.

Lest these contrasting portrayals be deemed caricatures, some 'softening' of their hard edges is needed. *First*, profiles of modal character do not rule out individual variability within a given society. Thus warm and friendly people with capacity for deep intimacy do exist in the West and cold, aloof and mistrustful ones in the East. Group tendencies painted with the broad brush of generalization must not be permitted to gloss over the finer nuances of individual psychodynamics. *Second*, both within the East and West, there might exist sub-cultural, regional and ethnic differences in the extent of interpersonal intimacy. For instance, the personal reserve deemed prototypical of White Anglo-Saxon Protestants ('WASPS') is not valid for African Americans or Italian Americans in the United States. And, in India, people of the states of Punjab and Tamil Nadu differ greatly in the extent of talkativeness, need for privacy and ease with which they make new friends. *Third*, economic class also plays a role here. Generally speaking, families of lower socioeconomic classes live in close proximity with each other. This necessitates greater interaction with relatives and with neighbors and other community members. Overcrowding within living quarters can lead to 'thinness' of personal boundaries and greater tolerance of intimacy. Even a cursory look at upper middle class, predominantly white, North American suburbs reveals the isolationism and crusty self-reliance of their inhabitants. Contact with neighbors is perfunctory and one sees fewer children playing outside the house. To paraphrase Freud's "anatomy is destiny" (1924, p. 178), observations such as these make one conclude that 'economy is destiny'. *Fourth*, a related variable pertains to rural vs. urban societies. The former provide great necessity and opportunity for close human relationships. The latter facilitate cloistered existence. Thus in rising world nations like China, Brazil and India, where rural to urban migration is occurring at an astounding pace (Akhtar, 2011), the shape and form of family units and modal child-rearing practices are also changing. These, in turn, might affect the personality attributes (including the capacity for intimacy) upheld as desirable and fitting for survival and progress. *Fifth*, one must not overlook that massive waves of migration are occurring from so-called Third World countries to the Western hemisphere. This provides a great opportunity for people of both regions to develop heteroethnic and homoethnic friendships. Elsewhere, I have elaborated on the differences and similarities of such bonds (Akhtar, 2011, pp. 81–102). Suffice here to say that in general, homoethnic friendships soothe and provide more intimate contact but can slow down individuation, whereas heteroethnic friendships propel acculturation and enrich culture-specific ego skills but preclude deeper intimacy. *Finally*, it should be remembered that the intimacy-privacy divide is not an 'all or none' phenomenon. It is not that Westerners need and value more privacy and Easterners need and value more intimacy. Both groups need and value both experiences. Their ways of obtaining these experiences might differ and the dramatis personae enlisted for important relationships might vary. More importantly, different layers of psychic structure might be used to achieve these goals. In this context, the astute observation of Roland (1988), a New York-based psychoanalyst with considerable clinical and social experience with Indian and Japanese clients and their respective homelands, is highly pertinent.

> As a counter to permeable outer ego boundaries in the intense familial intimacy relationships where there is little if any privacy, Indians establish another inner ego boundary to protect and enhance a highly private self with its rich feelings and fantasies – thus creating inner psychological space. This kind of ego boundary is as yet unformulated in psychoanalysis in the West – mainly because Western individualism, with its emphasis on strong outer ego boundaries and individual autonomy, precludes the necessity of developing such an inner boundary and private self as central psychological structures. (p. 227)

Endopsychic considerations such as these are useful reminders of the dialectical ties between anthropology and psychoanalysis (Paul, 2005) while also preparing the ground for us to re-enter the clinical realm. Before doing so, however, I will make a brief foray into some sub-optimally understood aspects of human intimacy.

Three unexplored realms of intimacy

Three areas, not widely recognized in the existing literature on intimacy, now draw my attention. Rendered as questions, these are: (i) Are there variable degrees of intimacy with one's different self-representations? (ii) Can intimacy exist between man and animal? (iii) Is there a sort of intimacy between a religious mendicant and his or her god? Allow me to make brief comments on each of these issues.

Intimacy with parts of oneself

A healthy and 'well-formed' self does not imply a monolithic homogeneity. In fact, a rigid and caricatured consistency is often a defense against internal divisions and chaos. A normal, well-integrated and smoothly functioning self is comprised of many subsets of self-representations (Eisnitz, 1980). Some of these are close to action, others to contemplation. Some are nearer to masculinity, others to femininity. Some express one life agenda, others a differing one. What distinguishes a cohesive self with multiple self-representations from a disordered identity is the former's overall synthesis, comfortable transition between various aspects, and an optimal mixture of reality principle and ego-ideal-dictated life direction in the manifestation or non-manifestation of this or that self-representation.

One might therefore maintain varying distances with different parts of one's self. Note here that Freud's topographic (1900) and structural (1923b) models of mind both permit a consideration of this sort and Bouvet (1958) who first wrote about 'optimal distance' was actually talking about "the gap that separates the way in which a subject expresses his instinctual drives from how he would express them if the process of 'handling' or 'managing' (in French: *amenagement*) these expression did not intervene" (p. 211, italics in the original). Besides such formal and dynamic separations, there are content-based divisions within the self. Bach's (1977) concept of 'mirror-complementarity of the self' whereby one consciously experienced and expressed behavioral extreme is almost always associated with its opposite (e.g. greed vs. generosity) refers to this very fact. So does Feldman's (2007) paper on the technique of addressing (or, not addressing) repudiated parts of the self during the analytic work.

Thus one's avowed self might maintain a close discourse with one self-representation and deny expression to another. I, for one, have avoided 'intimacy' with two aspects of myself: one pertains to gambling and the other to spirituality. Staying far from the former, I have not frequented casinos (after one mesmerizing trip to Atlantic City) and have never visited Las Vegas. Staying less distant from the latter, I have found promptings to renounce a well-chiselled selfhood alluring as well as frightening. I have flirted with desires to learn more about Buddhism and Sufism, to visit sacred places of the world, and to retreat into non-worldly solitude[9] but found such inner callings a bit scary. A gradual compromise on my part has been to read and write about human attributes such as forgiveness (Akhtar, 2002), goodness (Akhtar, 2009a, 2009b), gratitude (Akhtar, 2012a), generosity (Akhtar, 2012b), dignity (Akhtar, 2015), patience (Akhtar, 2015c) and humility (Akhtar, 2018). My lack of 'intimacy' with my gambler self has been good for me. My hesitation to fully encounter my 'spiritual self' (Roland, 2011) has produced ambivalent results. My own struggles notwithstanding, the question remains whether we – all of us can become 'intimate' with all parts of ourselves? And, if not, does such distance enrich or impoverish one's personality? Are compromises possible? And, do such compromises present themselves only in middle or old age or earlier as well?

Intimacy with animals

In *Totem and Taboo*, Freud (1913) famously declared that:

> Children show no trace of the arrogance which urges adult civilized men to draw a hard-and-fast line between their own nature and that of all other animals. Children have no scruples over allowing them to rank as their full equals. Uninhibited as they are in the avowal of their bodily needs, they no doubt feel themselves more akin to animals than to their elders, who may well be a puzzle to them.
>
> (pp. 126–127)

Four years later, Freud (1917) returned to this topic with the following statement:

> Man is not a being different from animals or superior to them; he himself is of animal descent, being more closely related to some species and more distantly to others. The acquisitions he has subsequently made have not succeeded in effacing the evidences, both in his psychic structure and mental dispositions, of his parity to them.
>
> (p. 141)

Freud's developmental theorizing emphasized the animal substrate of the inner world of human beings while also noting that animals frequently serve as symbolic reservoirs of our projections. Indeed, three out of his 'famous' four cases, namely those of Little Hans (1909b), the Rat Man (1909d) and Wolf Man (1918b), and involved human fantasies and preoccupations with animals.

This line of exploration in Freud's work was not advanced by later psychoanalysts, with the notable exception of Searles (1960) and, to a lesser extent, by Sperling (1952, 1971) and Shengold (1971). A major impetus was given to such conceptualization by two volumes that Volkan and I edited: *Mental Zoo* (Akhtar & Volkan, 2005a) and *Cultural Zoo* (Akhtar & Volkan, 2005b). We brought together a number of contemporary analysts who advanced Freud's preliminary notions about the role of domesticated or wild animals in the psychic development of a child; in his or her adaptation to the external world; and in the complex and rich tapestry of human culture including mythology, art, music, literature and cinema.

Now, taking a step towards deeper layers of man-animal relationship, I raise the question whether genuine intimacy can be a part of this bond. Putting aside the sexually perverse use of animals (Krafft-Ebing, 1892; Kinsey, Pomeroy, & Martin, 1948a, 1948b; Stolorow & Grand, 1973; Greenacre, 1951; Shengold, 1967; Traub-Werner, 1986) and cruelty towards them (Akhtar & Brown, 2005) where the relationship is exploitative, unempathic and one-sided, the answer to the question about genuine intimacy between man and animal seems to be affirmative. Experience with my pet dogs – Jackie and Majnun – my children's experiences with cats and horses, my observation of friends and patients who have owned pets, and my reading of novels involving man-animal relationship (e.g. Ackerley, 1956; Parkhurst, 2004) and newer psychoanalytic contributions (Bolognini, 2008; Platt, 2017) support such an assertion on my part.

All the components of intimacy – caring, trusting, sharing of experiences, discarding shame and facilitating the joyous expansion of the partner's self – can be found in man-animal relationship. The communication and exchange of such feelings occurs less on a verbal and more on a nonverbal, sensual and intuitive level. Writing specifically about the man-dog relationship, Bolognini (2008) declares that if the owner retains a "sufficiently liberated spirit" (p. 98) and can resist projecting his or her self-representations upon the animal partner, an "operative unity" (p. 99) and "shared directionality" (p. 105) between them can emerge; this can enrich both partners' emotional lives. I agree with this and add that we not only give all sort of nicknames to our animals, we also come up with nicknames we believe our pets have assigned to us. Such reciprocity is further enhanced by mutual play and respectful regard for each other's moods and state-related needs. Khan's (1983) observation that the presence of a dog in the house[10] can facilitate the master's 'lying fallow' is one shining example of the holding functions of man-animal relationships. Another illustration is contributed by the deeply affectionate mutuality between blind people and their seeing-eye dogs. The use of domesticated animals in nursing homes for the elderly is yet another example of the benefits of man-animal intimacy. More recently, the trust in horses' natural benevolence has been utilized to help crack the shell of impaired mentalization in autistic children (Murphy, 2011; Cahill, 2015), and to create confessional narratives that preclude recidivism for female prisoners nearing release from prison (Rellahan, 2017).

Intimacy with God

The dissolution of the self – or, at least, its partial dismantling – during the state of 'oceanic feeling' was attributed to transcendence by Rolland (letter to Freud, December 5, 1927; cited in Freud, 1930, p. 65) and to regression by Freud (1930). The sense that one is merged with the universe-at-large and all time and space is co-extensive with the ego was seen by the former as an arrival at a higher level of consciousness (where the self renounces its own boundaries) and was regarded by the latter as a return to an early infantile state (where the self is in a state of fusion with its surround, including, of course, the mother). With few exceptions (Rizzuto, 1979, 2001; Meissner, 1984, 2001), subsequent psychoanalysts followed Freud's line of thinking. They adapted his skeptical view of religious belief (Freud, 1927b) and helped create a heuristic atmosphere where psychoanalysis became a conjoined twin of atheism.

In light of this, most analysts might feel uneasy at my suggestion that intimacy can exist between man and God.[11] They might assert that since God is an imaginary creation of man and its existence merely intrapsychic, the question of intimacy with it should not even arise. To this objection, I respond by saying that if differing levels of intimacy can exist with different *self*-representations (as described above) then why not with different *object*-representations as well? Freud's (1927c) argumentative dismissal of God and the fervent advocacy of atheism by some contemporary thinkers (Hitchens, 2007; Dawkins, 2008; Thomson & Aukofer, 2011) cannot – indeed do not – rob people of the need to believe in a divine power and to carry on internal discourse with it. This 'divine internal object' (personal communication, Father Lee Makowski, January 21, 2001) or 'God representation' (Rizzuto, 2001) can acquire anthropomorphic attributes and content-specificity *or* it can be metaphorical and remain ensconced in the 'intermediate area of experience' (Winnicott, 1953). Projected outward, the former leads to idolatry and submission. Kept inside, the latter enhances gratitude and humility (Akhtar, 2018). My declaration that "God is a majestic poem" (Akhtar, 2009b, p. 5) is reflective of this latter stance. Needless to add that one can be informed by a poem and one can add further meanings and richness to it.

Seen this way, we are less surprised (than we would be if we got stuck in the futile debate whether God exists or does not exist) to find that alongside his vociferous claims to be an atheist, Freud paid repeated homage to God.

> Letters throughout Freud's life are replete with words and phrases such as "I passed my examinations with God's help"; "if God so wills"; "the good Lord"; "taking the Lord to task"; "into the keeping of the Lord"; "until after the Resurrection"; "science seems to demand the existence of God"; "God's judgement"; "God's will"; "God's grace"; "God above"; "if someday we meet above"; "in the next world"; "my secret prayer". In a letter to Oscar Pfister, Freud writes that Pfister was "a true servant of God" and was "in the fortunate position to lead others to God".
>
> (Nicholi, 2002, p. 51)

Clearly, Freud revolted against the externalized, stern, father-like God who demanded blind worship while fearlessly expressing humility towards the sublime object of wonder, awe and gratitude. Fascinatingly, in one of his last writings, Freud (1939) declared that believing in a universal God, typical of monotheistic religions, results in certain 'sacrifice of intimacy' (p. 128). To explain by caricature, one can say that the father of 12 children is less likely to be 'intimate' with each of his children than the father of one or two. This opens up the possibility that polytheistic religions which let their followers choose the deity to worship (e.g. male, female, child, animal, half-animal-half man and so on) might facilitate a greater intimacy between man and God. Hinduism, especially, offers "a transference pantheon" (Rao, 2005, p. 271) and with it, the possibility

> to create, through the plasticity afforded by polytheism, a God in one's very own image. This is exemplified by the common practice of *Ishta Devata* or a personal God of one's liking, a God that a family or family member adopts as personally significant beyond all the other Gods. The idea of choosing the

> form of God to worship or cherish is unique, but not unlike the practice of seeking the blessings of a Christian patron saint. . . . In India, Gods are transference Gods par excellence, one might go further and say that they are also gods of transference, meaning that in a fundamental way Hindu Gods extend themselves in turn as transformable beings and transference objects. They do so through the *Avatar* mechanism, usually translated as incarnation of descent (from a more exalted state), a cherished power of Hindu deities that allows for multiple lives, births, appearance, and attributes to suit temporal eras, social customs, and personal wishes.
>
> (pp. 291–292, italics in the original)

Such flexibility stands in sharp contrast to the paternal and paternalistic God of the three Abrahamic faiths. At the same time, softer forms of all these religions (e.g. Kabbalah of Judaism, various mystical sects of Christianity, Sufism of Islam) do permit a more playful and personal dialogue with God. This, in Ostow's (1995) terms, constitutes 'ultimate intimacy'.

Technical implications

Any consideration of the therapeutic implications of intimacy needs to begin by delineating the place such experience occupies in a given psychoanalytic therapy of human development. Two opposite conceptualizations exist. In the classical model (Freud, 1905a, 1915c), seeking release of instinctual tension is the main psychic motivator and the 'object' (that which will facilitate tension reduction) is secondary to the instinct's 'aim' (the particular tension which needs to be discharged). In the later emergent object relations model, "Libido is fundamentally object seeking" (Fairbairn, 1963, p. 224), attachment needs are supraordinate to instinctual gratification (Bowlby, 1958), and the child has an 'intimacy need' from the very beginning of his life (Sullivan, 1953). The classical perspective reluctantly permits the value of object specificity, but more on the level of experientially evolved wishes than on the level of hard-wired developmental needs. The object relations perspective emphasizes that fulfillment of intimacy need specifically involving the mother is essential to normal growth and development of the child. The two perspectives yield different therapeutic stances.

The classical perspective discourages intimacy with the patient. It advocates anonymity and abstinence on the therapist's part. Freud's use of the 'surgeon' and 'mirror' metaphors (1912e, pp. 115, 118) underscored the dispassionate and personally 'uninvolved' stance that he deemed optimal for the therapist to assume. While he acknowledged the "healing power of love" (1907, p. 22) and even said that "our cures are cures of love" (Freud, cited in Nunberg & Federn, 1962, p. 101), officially, he recommended that the doctor "should be opaque to this patients" (1912e, p. 118) and must avoid giving personal information or even a glimpse of his feelings to the patient. Admonitions of this sort encouraged subsequent analysts to adopt a remote and distant stance from the patient's subjective emotionality. A tragic limit was reached when Hartmann (1960) declared that "analytic therapy is a kind of technology" (p. 21). Thus was born a 'non-relational' or what I call 'motherless' psychoanalysis.

Disagreements with such pseudo-scientific austerity were evident from the earlier days of psychoanalysis. Ferenczi (1928, 1931) placed emotional contact between the analyst and the patient at the center of what was therapeutic about psychoanalysis. And, his attitude was reflected in the later writings of his pupil, Balint (1953, 1968). In the United States, it is the organizationally side-lined and academically unsung Sullivan (1953) who championed this cause. He emphasized that the human need for emotional contact with others is innate and the failure to meet this need leads to disorganization in childhood and loneliness in adult life. Sullivan's notion of treatment included the therapist's becoming, by his very warmth and humanity, a useful presence that transcends transferential fantasy and satisfies the need for intimacy. Representing this way of thinking, Ferreira (1964) stated that "in psychotherapy, it is not the explanation but the experience that counts" (p. 193). Developing the proposal further, Levenson (1974) declared that all interpretations are, in the end, acts of countertransference. The analyst "must not use himself as a tool to lever the patient into change" (p. 365). An additional feature to such therapeutic approach is for the analyst to share something subjective of himself with the patient. In Hirsch's (1983) words, "The exposure of the self of the analyst and the self of the patient reflects analytic intimacy" (p. 327). The analyst's resonating with the patient's experience and helping him find more nuances of it within himself is what is therapeutic about psychoanalysis. This is what I term the 'fatherless' version of psychoanalytic technique.

This classical-relational divide has had many incarnations, beginning with Freud-Ferenczi disagreements through the Klein-Balint schism, down to the current tension between the 'modern ego psychology' and relational, intersubjective approaches to technique. The names keep changing and lineages are highlighted or denied[12], but issues remain the same. The technical impacts of this divergence are too extensive to cover here, and we need to keep a tight focus on the issue of intimacy.

In the classical technique, the demand for free association 'forces' the patient to reveal his fantasies and secrets while the analyst remains 'opaque'. This does not seem to qualify as intimacy especially if the mutuality and bilaterality are held as its central ingredients. How can the patient be intimate if the analyst is reserved? In the relational technique, the subjective experience of the patient is regarded as always valid and a shared responsiveness and openness in the clinical dyad is recommended. The therapist is discouraged from ascribing greater significance to his understanding of the patient's experience. Kohut (1977) and Schwaber (2007) both support such 'anti-interpretation posture', though from differing theoretical bases. Nosek (2009) is even more vocal in this regard.

> If we are prepared to forgo the violence of knowledge, if we are not incited by the urgency of ontology and the power of positivism, we encounter the territory of hospitality; this means receiving the foreigner as such, allowing him his own existence. This gesture, configured as goodness, does not ennoble or exalt me; its character comes from the infinite to be received, unravelling my

> possibilities. . . . For us psychoanalysts, this is a radical hierarchical reflection; psychoanalysis is no longer a talking cure but a listening cure.
>
> (p. 145)

Levenson (1974) seeks a compromise position by saying that "after the experience of the patient and therapist has been validated, a content interpretation has the value of supplying the patient with a coherent myth, an armature on which to hang the story" (p. 365). Giving a little more credit to the usefulness of interpretation, I have noted how the analyst needs to oscillate with the ebb-and-flow of his patient's material, making validating comments at one moment, and deciphering interventions at another (Akhtar, 2002).

The temptation here is to regard the intimacy born out of intersubjective attunement and interpretation derived from 'objective listening' (Akhtar, 2013a) as separate entities. The fact, however, is that an interpretative element is always embedded in the most affirmative of analyst's remarks. The following three vignettes exemplify this assertion.[13]

Clinical vignette: I

Andrea Hooberman, a 55-year-old divorced and childless schoolteacher, was in the clutches of deep anguish when she sought my help. A botched surgical operation had recently left her with a dysfunction that made it impossible for her to enjoy sex. She had also become fecally incontinent. Multiple consultations with physicians and surgeons confirmed that the damage was irreversible. While she had sued the original surgeon and was expecting a huge monetary settlement, this hardly consoled her.

In her work with me, Andrea would often break down and weep bitterly. Once, pulling herself out of such emotional flooding, she looked at me intently and asked: "So, what are *you* thinking?" Without a moment's delay, I responded: "Actually, I was having two thoughts. One, I want to find you a great surgeon who can fix your problem. And, two, I am thinking how can I kill you painlessly to relieve you of this unbearable suffering". Andrea looked at me, nodded, and mumbled: "Thank you".

Clinical vignette: 2

Lisa Fischetti, a 22-year-old college student, was in treatment with me for a long-term sense of inferiority, inability to say 'no' and doubt about her self-worth. She came across as charming, intelligent and witty, but felt that she had little to offer and would be of no interest to anyone worthwhile. The two things she acknowledged to be good in her life were her academic performance and the fact that she had developed a good friendship with her roommate. And then one day, a disaster happened: this friend of hers was run over by a drunk driver and died on the spot. Lisa was devastated.

In the session immediately following this accident, Lisa cried and cried: her body curled up in pain, her face wet with tears, her sobs and wails filling up the psychic space between us. I remained mostly silent till almost the end of the session when I said: "You know, being an analyst, I am not permitted to do certain things. Had I not been bound by such ethics, I would have gotten up from my chair and given you a long and tight hug". Lisa looked up, met my eyes, and nodded with understanding and gratitude.

Clinical vignette: 3[14]

Katherine O'Malley had lost her mother to lung cancer at the age of 4 and a half. Although her father was very loving, her stepmother's duty-bound, anti-instinctual and humorless attitude left Katherine with a life-long wound of maternal loss. She achieved great success in her profession, married and raised two kids but always felt that something was missing from her life; a gnawing anguish persisted. This became worse when her teenage daughter got into drugs. Katherine now entered analysis and was surprised to discover the pervasive, even if subtle, effects of the childhood maternal loss upon her psychosocial functioning. Grieving that had been 'deferred' (Freud, 1918b) now began in earnest and occupied center stage for the first two years of her analysis.

In the fourth year, when such mourning seemed to have subsided, a disturbing external event re-kindled the grief. Katherine was overwhelmed and began crying profusely during one session. Barely able to stop heaving and sobbing, she said, "I thought it was over but surely, it is not". I felt moved to respond and said, "You know, two lines from a poem in my mother-tongue came to mind in response to what you just said. I know you will not understand them but let me recite them first and then I will translate them for you". After this, I recited, "*Kitne toofaN uthhaye aankhoN ne // Naao yaadoN ki doobti; hi nahiN*" //[15] I then paused and said, "It means that how many, just how many storms my eyes have borne but this goddamn boat of memory never sinks". Feeling understood and well 'held', Katherine nodded and became calmer.

As would be readily evident, these vignettes have many elements in common. In all three instances, the patient was in the throes of powerful emotions and I was correspondingly moved. In all three instances, I made a certain kind of self-disclosure (in the first, of a fantasy I was having; in the second, of an act I would have performed were it not a clinical situation; and in the third, of my need to speak in my mother tongue that was not comprehensible to the patient). In all three instances, there was a marked authenticity and a spontaneity to my intervention. In all three instances, the patient's response to my intervention was feeling deeply understood.

Together these features make such interventions appear akin to what Bion (1970) has called 'acts of faith'; these refer to interventions that arise from a sudden intuition which, for one shining moment, has left all prior experience and knowledge behind. This is true if we focus on my speaking alone. However, if we pay attention to the relational matrix of these vignettes, then Stern et al.'s (1998) 'moments of meeting' seem a more apt designation. A 'moment of meeting' is "a newly created dyadic state . . . [and] the point at which the intersubjective context gets altered" (p. 913). Stern et al. emphasize that interpretations can lead to a 'moment of meeting' and a 'moment of meeting' can lead to an interpretation.[16] I agree and add that comments made during such moments carry both affirmative-validating and interpretative-unmasking elements in them.

Thus in the first vignette, my comment not only resonated with the helplessness of the patient, it also unmasked the temptation towards omnipotence under such circumstances. Similarly, in the second vignette, my comment demonstrated that I was aware of how upset that patient was while simultaneously deciphering the ordinary human desire for being comforted during grief. Finally, in the third vignette, the choice of the poetic piece was in attunement with the patient's suffering while the use of my mother tongue conveyed that I myself was less 'empty' and could offer her maternal nourishment. To go back to a comment I made in the developmental section of this paper, both 'maternal intimacy' and 'paternal intimacy' were at work in unison. This, to my mind, erases the sharp distinction between offering intimacy and making an interpretation, thus bridging a schism that has long existed in our theory of technique.

Conclusion

In this contribution, I have surveyed the psychoanalytic literature on the concept of intimacy. From this review, I have culled seven components of intimacy, including trust, sharing of private experiences and feelings, relaxation of boundaries, overcoming of personal shame, empathy, tenderness and transcendence of gender boundaries. I have discussed the developmental prerequisites for the capacity for such intimacy, emphasizing the role played by early maternal attunement to the child's needs and emotions and by the mother's ability to bear some distance from the child and encourage individuation. I have noted that the refinement of the capacity for intimacy occurs in latency and adolescence and true intimacy is achieved by the merger of affection and sexuality at the onset of young adulthood.

Following this, I have delineated four psychopathological derailments of this capacity: (i) failed intimacy, (ii) florid intimacy, (iii) fluctuating intimacy and (iv) false intimacy. Then I have delved into the sociocultural realm as it pertains to the form, extent and purview of intimacy. And, finally, I have elucidated the place of intimacy in the analytic situation, providing a few clinical illustrations that highlight the analyst's participation in such moments of deep contact.

Before concluding this discourse, I must add that in healthy individuals the capacity for intimacy is not compulsively deployed. It is under voluntary control; one can chose to be intimate with one person and not with another. One can also regulate the velocity of such development. Moreover, the capacity of intimacy does not preclude the ability to relate with others in a non-intimate manner. Even with one's lover, the degree of intimacy undergoes ebb and flow. In this vein and coming back full circle to where I started from, I conclude this contribution with another of my father's *shers* (couplets) which notes that the beloved who has become truly certain of the lover's devotion can become free, at times, to be lovingly indifferent towards him. The actual words of my father (J.N. Akhtar, 1964, p. 32) are:

Aitmaad-e-mohabbat to dekhe koi
Un meiN ik khaas begaana-pun aagaya.

Notes

1 Such literal translation of these couplets has resulted in a regrettable loss of their prosodic beauty. I therefore feel sorry for all three parties involved here – the poet, myself as an amateur translator and the reader – for this loss.

2 A related question in today's world is whether intimacy – romantic or friendly – can be developed and sustained via electronic communication systems such as Skype, FaceTime and Instant Chat applications. The knee-jerk reaction of skepticism regarding such relationships is rapidly becoming old-fashioned. People are carrying on all sorts of meaningful dialogues with each other on such social media: business-related, familial, romantic, erotic, bullying and sexually perverse. Some of these contacts do qualify as 'intimate'. Psychoanalytically biased idealization of personal contact may be hard to justify when we learn of well-meaning and distinguished colleagues conducting analytic treatments across nations and continents. To refute that they are involved in an intimate discourse is to take a position that is becoming less defensible in the contemporary world, although, as the authors in Chapter 8 argue, there may well be elements that are lost in digital translation.

3 Kafka's (1989) concept of the 'primary paradox of individuation' also touches upon this matter. According to him, healthy mother-child symbiosis permits the child to grow and step away from its mother. In such a setting, "love and mutual acceptance of separateness become subjectively equivalent" (p. 33).

4 A striking example of friendly intimacy was recently related by one of my supervisees. She was invited by a close friend of hers to be present in the labor room as the latter delivered her first child. The friend's husband was also present there but since neither the friend nor her husband had medical backgrounds, the invitation to a physician friend provided healthy rationalization to what, at its depth, might have carried complex emotional motives. On the other hand, this gesture might have simply been

a testimonial to friendly intimacy (Ariela Green, personal communication, December 21, 2017).

5 My proposal contains an echo of Herzog's (1984) homeostatic and disruptive attunements, i.e. maternal provision of validity and harmony, and paternal nudge towards self-expansion.

6 I have elsewhere (Akhtar, 2018) elucidated the concept of humility in considerable detail.

7 Freud and Jung, who reported talked incessantly for 13 continuous hours upon meeting each other for the first time (Gay, 1988) unfortunately did not do so well in the long run.

8 Like the proverbial 'return of the repressed', childhood keeps making ferocious claims upon the daily lives of adult Americans. The sight of people carrying water bottles with eyes fixed on their iPhone screens 'confirms' the continued oral-visual cathexis of the maternal breast. Vestimentary distinction between children and adults is blurred. Blockbuster movies center upon superheroes, magical settings and animation – all staples of children's imagination. And, television commercials are replete with animal (actually, animated) spokesmen pushing this or that merchandise. Together, such cultural phenomena reflect a desperate clinging to childhood among people who have not had their fill when they really were children.

9 Much to the disbelief of friends to whom I have told this, I was utterly fascinated by (and wanted to follow the lead of) Carmelite mendicants who take a vow of silence and spend their lives in cloistered prayer. More recently, my seeing the photographs of the 4th-century Sumela monastery in Turkey had a similarly alluring effect upon me.

10 While Khan does not specify it, my sense is that it needs a big dog to facilitate the owner's lying fallow. Most small dogs are too frisky and playful to provide such a holding function.

11 The fact is that a large number of books exist that are titled *Intimacy with God* (e.g. Heald, 2000; Keating, 2009; Jakes, 2013; Oberto, 2017).

12 For various 'political' reasons, the current relational analysts do not declare that their conceptual and theoretical ancestry goes back to Sullivan.

13 The names given to patients in these vignettes are fictitious.

14 This case has also been included elsewhere (Akhtar, 2015) in a different context.

15 The line comes from a poem by the contemporary Urdu poet of India, Akhlaq Mohammad Khan Shahryar (1936–2012).

16 Yerushalmi (2013) has noted that theoretical developments encouraging analysts to create such moments increase the risk of countertransference enactments.

The spectrum of intimacy

Chapter 2

Attachment and intimacy

April Fallon and Rama Rao Gogineni

Intimacy, love and compassion are overlapping and intertwined aspects of the human experience that develop through the lifespan. The ability and ease in giving and receiving these experiences enhances one's quality of physical and social life or potentially destines one to loneliness, alienation and despair (Durkheim, Buss, Sennett, & Riley, 1897). The underpinnings of these capacities can be understood within the framework of the attachment and caregiving systems which have evolutionary foundations and are formed and reworked throughout a lifetime (Bowlby, 1969, 1973, 1980, 1988). In this chapter we focus on how attachment and caregiving affect the capacity and desire for intimacy in adults, weaving theory, research and clinical observation. We briefly review the origins of the attachment bonds and caregiving systems. We then highlight research and provide brief clinical examples that illustrate how differences in attachment affect the development of intimacy and relationships.

Constructs of intimacy, attachment and caregiving

Intimacy

While 'intimacy' came into use as a euphemism for sexual intercourse in the 1600s, its meaning has broadened in contemporary use (Online Etymology Dictionary, 2018; Random House, 2018). 'Intimate' refers to private and personal (Dictionary.com, 2018). The Latin, *intimus*, translates into the "inmost, profound most or very secret" (Wiktionary, 2018). We are most interested in it as it applies to the relational domain – the close, familiar and usually affectionate or loving personal connection with another person. Intimacy may involve a mental, physical (including affectionate and sexual), social and/or emotional closeness. Intimate relationships encompass physical, emotional, social, intellectual, spiritual and recreational dimensions (Bochner, 2017). Adult intimacy involves the knowledge and acceptance of one's private feelings and behaviors, the sharing of it truthfully with another and accepting of the other's inner good and bad characteristics, conscious and unconscious. We explore how the capacity for intimacy is significantly influenced by the development of early attachment bonds. Cassidy (2001) has articulated four essential abilities required for intimacy that can be viewed as emerging from the primary caregiver's sensitive care and the ensuing quality of attachment that the child develops – the ability to seek out care, the ability to give care, the ability to feel comfortable with an autonomous self and the ability to negotiate. These will be further elaborated upon after the constructs of attachment and caregiving are described.

Attachment theory

Proposed by Bowlby (1958) and empirically supported by Ainsworth (1967), attachment theory is ensconced in an ethological and Darwinian evolutionary framework. The essence of it proposes that infants have an inborn propensity to seek and develop a unique and enduring affectional bond in order to increase their chances of survival. To that end, the infant is equipped with an innate and developing repertoire of behaviors (e.g. crying, smiling) that are likely to provoke caregiving in a maternally sensitive adult (Bowlby, 1958).[1] These behaviors become increasingly sophisticated and interactive as the infant matures and the caregiver becomes more engaged and attuned to the child idiosyncrasies.[2] The child's desire for proximity varies depending upon the child's age, internal state (e.g. if sick or hungry) and the perceived environmental threats. Bowlby describes the attachment system as one of several biologically based regulatory behavioral systems that are in dynamic equilibrium to each other. These other systems mature over the course of development as well. The exploratory system allows the child to explore the world and increases survival. When the child experiences the maternal connection as providing both a safe haven and a 'secure base', the need for attachment behaviors is downregulated; play and exploration increase. The fear system, aroused by frightening environmental stimuli, increases survival and also activates attachment seeking and deactivates exploratory behaviors. The sociable or affiliative behavioral system promotes proximity to peers and fosters the development of social skills and other non-attachment affectional bonds. The sociability behavioral system is activated when the attachment and fear systems are not (Cassidy, 2016).

There is a preference for a principal attachment figure, most frequently the biological mother initially, which is referred to as 'monotrophy' (Bowlby, 1969).[3] When separated involuntarily from the attachment figure, the child experiences distress and seeks proximity, security and comfort in that primary attachment (Bowlby, 1973, 1980). If the separation persists, the initial distress and protest become despair and finally detachment. The ontogeny of attachment bonds over the first four years of life have significant influence over the development of trust, emotion regulation, social skills, positive identity and quality of relationships throughout the lifespan (Marvin, Brittner, & Russell, 2016; Mikulincer & Shaver, 2016).[4]

Attachment bonds are co-constructed in the mother-child relationship. A child, with unique biological proclivities, and the attachment figure engage in a multitude of daily sensory, physical and verbal interactions which transform over the course of the preschool years. In normal development, the relationship proceeds from the necessity of physical proximity to the primary attachment to a more symbolic enduring "representation in the internal organization of the individual" (Ainsworth, 1989, p. 711). Bowlby referred to this internalized relationship as an 'internal working model' and outlines four stages of development. The first, which lasts from birth to approximately 3 months, entails the infant gazing, crying, grasping and smiling, with the mother returning loving gazes, touching, holding and sensitively meeting biological needs and required level of comfort. In the second phase, which ends at approximately 6–9 months, the child focuses increasingly more elaborate behaviors toward familiar caregivers with differentiated vocalizations, gestures and exploratory behavior (Ainsworth, 1967). The quality of attachment is affected by the "extent to which the mother has permitted clinging, and following, and all the behaviors associated with them" (Bowlby, 1958, p. 370). The next stage, from 6 to 9 months up to 18 months–2 years, involves the child's increased locomotion and burgeoning cognitive development which allows for interactions to become symbolic. The key component – a felt security – is the child's notion of where the attachment figures can be found if needed and how the child expects them to respond. Bowlby (1969) notes, "The mothers whose infants are more securely attached to them are mothers who respond to their babies' signals promptly and appropriately, and who engage in much social interchange with them – to the delight of each party" (p. 316). At the same time, there is increased fear and wariness toward unfamiliar people. Bowlby observed that a significant disruption of this bond between mother and child after one-year mark increases the possibility of long-term negative outcomes. Research on adoption confirms that those children adopted after their first year of life are more likely to suffer from reactive attachment disorders and increased insecure attachment styles, whereas those adopted before 1 year of age appear similar to the cohort of biological children.[5] The child's physical, cognitive and emotional growth allows for greater flexibility in how felt security is maintained. At this stage, the child develops more stable sociable, attachment, fear and exploratory behavioral systems and preferred strategies to manage attachment needs become more salient. In the final stage, from 18 months to 2 years and on, a goal-corrected partnership is achieved where both mother and child negotiate a mutual plan for proximity (Bowlby, 1969). The children recognize that others have thoughts that are distinct from theirs. The perceived availability of the primary attachment figure rather than physical connection is the central component in security experienced. Although the child's temperament, biology and environmental circumstances are important, the quality and variations in attachment capacities are significantly influenced by the sensitivity and caregiving of the attachment figure(s) (Bowlby, 1973; Kobak, Zajac, & Madsen, 2016).

Early research by Ainsworth (1954, 1985) first observing families with infants and then later developing the strange situation procedure distinguished three specific strategies that toddlers used in dealing with separation and have come to represent types of attachment that children were observed to have: secure, avoidant and ambivalent attachment. How children interacted with parents during play and exploration, how they reacted to brief separations from and then reunion with the attachment figure, and how they respond to a stranger's affiliative efforts differed among the three types. Securely attached children were distressed when their mothers left but were calmed by the mother's return. These children were interested in their environment when the attachment figure was present. The avoidant group of children appeared relatively undisturbed when the mother left and did not reunite with her when she returned. The anxious ambivalent group was distressed when their mothers left. When their mothers returned they seemed to want comfort, but rejected bids by the mother to do so, continuing to express distress. These children are reluctant to explore their environment even when mother is present. Main and Solomon (1990) added a disorganized style where the child's exhibited conflicting behaviors, alternating between approaching the mother and freezing upon reunion. The Adult Attachment Interview was developed as an alternative method with adults to mirror the strange situation for children (George, Kaplan, & Main, 1985). Adult memories of their primary attachment figures are evaluated for coherence and integration. To understand attachment in the child more fully, we introduce the complementary maternal caregiving system and discuss the relationship between caregiving and the child's attachments.

The caregiving system

Attachment initially was conceptualized as the child's connection to the primary caregiver (Bowlby, 1969). The caregiving behavioral system is the complementary response of the caregiver's sensitivity and effectiveness in providing a safe haven (safety from danger, access to comfort for the distress) and a secure base (support for exploring the world and promoting the psychological and social growth) for the child. Ainsworth (1985) in her research with Baltimore and Ugandan mothers found that attachment figures who responded promptly and sensitively encouraged attachment security with their children. Meta-analyses have confirmed the link between maternal sensitivity, maternal attachment and child attachment security (DeWolff & Van Ijzendoorn, 1997; Van Ijzendoorn, 1995). Similarly, a meta-analysis of father sensitivity is modestly but significantly linked to child attachment (Lucassen et al., 2011).[6] The intergenerational transmission of these relationships cannot be explained by genetics (Feeney & Woodhouse, 2016).[7]

In addition to consistency and responsivity, what aspects of caregiving are more specifically responsible for this link to child attachment? Reviewing the research, Solomon and George (2008) posit that coherence, balance and flexibility of the maternal caregiver impact attachment bonds. Children securely connected to their mothers are more likely to have representations of mothers who are flexible and coherent. In contrast, insecurely attached children have disparate, unintegrated and hostile representations of their mothers. Bowlby (1980) characterizes the underlying processes for these differences as a result of mothers' unconscious methods of processing relational connections and related memories.

These defenses are "an exclusion from further processing of information of certain specific types for relatively long periods or even permanently" (p. 45). There are three forms of exclusion: deactivation, cognitive disconnection and segregation (Bowlby, 1980; Solomon & George, 2008).

Mothers who use deactivation manage anxieties about safety and loss in the relationship by diminishing the importance of the relational connection, even when children are under 1 year of age. Although these mothers may be consistent, responsible and view themselves as caring, they often oversee their children from a psychological distance. For example, when a mother of a 2-month-old decided to return to work which involved much time away from home, she reasoned the father and grandmother could provide for the child in her absence. She planned elaborate schedules and made lists of tasks that needed to be done, yet seemed to have little thought about the child missing her or her missing the child. These mothers encourage early exploration and value the child's accomplishments such as talking. Mothers who use this relational strategy extensively often have children with avoidant attachment style. When mothers use cognitive disconnection their affect and the events they experience are disconnected; neither is completely remembered or excluded. In contrast to mothers who use deactivation, these mothers provide close physical and psychological oversight and cannot separate themselves from their child's psychological or physical discomforts.

They often express intense anxiety over the child's safety and their lack of control over it and externalize their anger toward outsiders. Mothers who use this strategy extensively have children who are fearful of exploration and often have anxious ambivalent attachment styles. For example, a pediatrician referred a mother whose infant was dehydrated and emaciated. This seemed to be the result of mother producing very little milk, but refusing to give supplements, blaming the lactation consultants for not providing more assistance. Breast feeding was extremely important to her sense of competence as a mother. She did not recognize the danger that her child was in. She would also not allow the father or relatives to hold the infant or help care for the infant, afraid that they would drop the baby.

A use of 'segregated defenses' is the most pathological and often the result of a mother's traumas that are either unconscious or conscious. These intrude into her thoughts and overwhelm her so that she cannot adequately attend to her baby's needs, leaving the child vulnerable to a disorganized attachment and at risk for later more severe psychopathology (Solomon & George, 2008). Fraiberg et al. (1975) provide some excellent examples of these mothers.

Research on this topic has revealed two other prominent factors in the development of healthy attachments. The first is the caregiver's 'mind-mindedness', which is the recognition that the child has a mind separate from the caregiver (Meins et al., 2012). Sensitively knowing the child deeply and respecting the child's separateness provide a model for later empathic accuracy of another. Second, the primary caregiver's avoidance of closeness (eye gaze, smiling, holding, cuddling, etc.) and a decreased display of emotions are linked to less sensitive and responsive caregiving. This early avoidance and lack of physical and emotional connection sets up a working model of adult relationships that lacks in intimate behaviors. Over the course of development, mothers and other caregivers are not perfect. Most children tolerate some parental insensitivity as long as major caregivers are not hostile or frightening and could reasonably manage the attachment-exploration balance. That is, major caregivers can be intrusive and insensitive as long as their intrusiveness does not activate the child's attachment system (Feeney & Woodhouse, 2016). It has been shown that therapy and even brief interventions that improve parental sensitivity augment children's attachment security (Bakermans-Kranenburg, Van Ijzendoorn, & Juffer, 2003).

Caregiving abilities are a function of having been cared for. Physical, emotional and instrumental support enhances psychological wellbeing by providing a safe environment when children are distressed (safe haven) and supporting their personal growth with a safety net to fall back upon (secure base). Effective caregiving determines the quality of the attachment bond between child and mother and impacts the child's ability to become a future caregiver to progeny, as well as the capacity for romantic and other affectional bonds.

As Freud has suggested, psychic structures and behaviors likely have biological foundations. Nascent research in neurobiology has suggested that two neuro endocrine systems, oxytocinergic and dopaminergic, have been implicated in attachment and maternal caregiving. The former is important in the formation of social memories, affiliative behavior and emotional regulation (Diminich & Bonanno, 2014; Strathearn, 2011). The latter is involved in the reward system. There is new work (mostly in animal models) that suggests that the release of oxytocin, a neuropeptide by the posterior pituitary hormone, is implicated in the maternal bond.[8] Toward the end of pregnancy, oxytocin has been found to increase and then surge after birth in new mothers. It aids the childbirth process and helps with nursing. In response to social cues, it also has been found to activate the dopaminergic reward system which may help explain the intense pleasure that mothers experience with their newborns. These two systems likely interconnect with the infant's vocalization and tactile stimulation, releasing oxytocin which may result in the activation of the dopaminergic reward pathway. In addition, oxytocin appears to have long-term anxiolytic effects. Women who report emotional neglect in childhood have lower levels of oxytocin, and mothers who neglect their infants also appear to have lower indicators of oxytocin. Individuals with insecure and dismissing attachment have both a reduced activation of the dopamine reward system when viewing infant faces and decreased oxytocin in response to mother-infant contact (Strathearn, 2011). There is also a correlation between mother-infant oxytocin levels. Oxytocin also increases in fathers, but not until after birth. Thus it appears that oxytocin increases mothers' and fathers' caregiving behaviors which are rewarding and thus reinforcing. These in turn match the infant's affiliative and pleasure neurobiological systems (Bretherton & Munholland, 2016). Caregiving impacts attachment and attachment then influences the next generation of caregiving. These systems are likely biologically primed and unfold differentially with critical environmental events.

Attachment from the cradle to the grave

Bowlby (1969) distinguishes attachment bonds from other social relationships with defining features of safe haven, proximity maintenance, separation distress and secure base. Affectional bonds are emotional connections to a specific person who does not necessarily provide protection, but satisfies humans' needs for social connection. Initially all later relationships were viewed as affectional. However, in Bowlby's (1988) later work, he suggested: "All of us, from the cradle to the grave, are happiest when life is organized as a series of excursions . . . from the secure base provided by our attachment figures" (p. 62). Burgeoning research on romantic partners has suggested that not only do these pair bonds function as attachment figures, but there is an evolutionary adaptation to this connection (Zeifman & Hazan, 2016). As the child grows, there are three changes in attachment from the early primary attachment bond. First, the necessity of proximity gradually is replaced by a mental representation. Second, the touch prominent in early attachments gradually includes sexual intimacy during adolescence and early adulthood. Third, the asymmetry of the care is replaced by a more reciprocal mutual security and caregiving expectations and behaviors.

While parents continue to provide a base for security through much of adolescence, between 8 and 14 years of age, children prefer peers to parents for emotional support. Most adults prefer peers to parents for support and safety. However, a fully formed adult attachment bond is more than simply preference for support; it takes time to develop the primacy that the maternal bond had. Neuroimaging studies support that brain activation in early relationships involves the dopamine system, whereas those in romantic relationships longer than two years, there is activation in the opioid regions associated with maternal attachment (Acevedo, Aron, Fisher, & Brown, 2012). The physical touch between a mother and child broadens to include intimate sexual contact in adults, the latter of which generates a surge of oxytocin for both men and women. This suggests that repeated intimate and sexual contact promotes the development of attachment in adults (Young & Wang, 2004). The primary attachment between parent and child becomes redirected in adolescence and adulthood toward a longer term sexual partner. Love and intimacy activate the same neural pathways as does attachment (Fischer, Aron, Mashek, Strong, Li, & Brown, 1998). Losses, such as death, have the same components as what early attachment loss exhibits (Fraley & Shaver, 2016). Romantic relationships of greater than two years (often referred to as pair-bonding) can contain the four essential components of attachment (proximity maintenance, separation distress, safe haven and secure base) that the primary infant-mother attachment bond exhibits (Fraley & Davis, 1997; Fraley & Shaver, 2000; Zeifman & Hazen, 2016).[9] Zeifman and Hazen (2016) argue and provide empirical evidence to support their notion that long-term bonds contribute to the survival and reproductive fitness of their offspring, as well as increase physical and mental health for the pair. When long-term bonds are secure, there are multiple advantages throughout the lifespan (Ainsworth, 1989; Bowlby, 1969, 1988).

How early attachment affects the development of adult intimacy

The relationship of attachment to intimacy suggests that early attachments form the basis for quality of later romantic relationships and the expression of intimacy (Mayseless & Scharf, 2007). Neuroimaging studies suggest that in adult relationships, intimacy and attachment overlap considerably in dopaminergic and oxytocin systems activated. When these are not activated, we see poorer quality of both attachment and lower levels of intimacy achieved. Beginning in adolescence, sexuality is linked to intimacy and attachment. There is evidence that sexual activity fosters adult attachment; oxytocin, involved in the maternal bond, surges in males and females during orgasm and relationships that evolve into attachment bonds are those in which there is heightened physiological arousal. An attachment bond to a sexual partner keeps the couple together and increases the chances of survival because both will protect the offspring.

Early attachment bonds impact subsequent sexual behavior and competence. It has been found that securely attached adults are less likely to be involved in one-night stands, report being involved in mutually satisfying sexual activity and enjoy physical contact. In contrast anxiously attached women report greater exhibitionism, voyeurism and dominance-bondage, and anxiously attached males are more reticent in their sexual activity. Avoidant adults report less enjoyment of physical contact, more one-night stands and more sexual contact outside the primary relationship (Cassidy, 2001).

In the internal working model, mental representations of the self and self-in-relationship to important others can affect the individual's interest and capacity in intimate relationships. A wanting to be with, the desire to know another deeply, to share one's self, to have the capacity to be comforted by another are important aspects of an intimate relationship. Secure attachment is associated with the capacity for intimacy in the following six domains: (i) the wish to be in an intimate relationship, (ii) the reasonable and accurate perception of its intensity, (iii) the ability and interest in obtaining care from others, (iv) giving care to others, (v) feeling comfort with one's autonomous self and (vi) the ability to negotiate differences (Cassidy, 2001).

Perception and assessment of closeness

A research study with married couples found that those with secure attachment are comfortable with intimacy, more readily trust and report greater marital satisfaction than those with less secure attachment (Feeney, 1996). Those preoccupied and fearful depended upon others for self-worth, worried intensely about their relationships and were dissatisfied with the closeness they experienced. Secure individuals tend to pair with other secure individuals, and those with secure attachments are more likely to experience intimacy in relationships (Bartholomew, 1990).

Attachment theory suggests that intimate relationships form through the lens of early mother-child attachment experience. This enables a securely attached individual to perceive someone as compatible and co-create a relational dynamic that provides safety and comfort and allows for growth (Ren, Arriaga, & Mahan, 2017). A large internet survey of 150,000 participants concretized how people define and perceive intimacy and sought to link it to attachment styles (Hudson & Fraley, 2017). The investigators found that highly anxious individuals have greater requirements for what constitutes a close relationship than those with secure attachment; they require more time, affection and self-disclosure to call a relationship 'close'. In contrast, those with high avoidance desire lower affection, less time and less self-disclosure to perceive a relationship as intimate. In this study, vignettes of high and low intimacy were presented and participants rated how close they perceived them. Those with anxious attachment perceived individuals as less close than did secure individuals. Higher avoidance individuals perceived the vignettes as more close. These differences were more exaggerated for those vignettes designed to depict lower levels of closeness.

This study suggests that highly anxious individuals want more closeness and are less likely to recognize closeness than those who are less anxious. Avoidant people require less time, affection and self-disclosure to define a relationship as close and perceive more closeness in the relationship vignettes than actually existed. This study demonstrated that attachment avoidance and anxiety influence the criteria that each feels represents 'close' behavior and bias the perception of intimacy. This is consistent with other research (Pietromonaco & Beck, 2015) that suggests that people have attentional biases and reconstruct memories that are consistent with their preferred strategies of affect regulation (Dykas & Cassidy, 2011). That is, insecure individuals compared to those more secure are more likely to remember negative events and interpret these events as more relationship threatening.

Clinical vignette: I

Mark and Joanna demonstrate these differences in attachment and intimacy. Both of them had been in individual therapy for several years when it seemed that conflict in their ten-year marriage increased beyond what they could tolerate. Mark was a professional and worked long hours. Joanna worked part time and had the majority of the child care responsibilities for their two young children. Mark was unhappy with their sex life, the amount of time he spent with his wife and their overall level of intimacy. He wanted some contact during the day – "an occasional call or text". Joanna felt too busy, too thinly stretched, and did not see need for this kind of connection. She felt that his demands were too intense, given her job and responsibilities with the children and house. She felt too tired for sex during the week. When Mark would come home, late in the evening, Joanna, having just settled the children, would be watching TV or be on the phone with friends. He felt angry that she would choose those activities over talking with him. There were occasional screaming arguments between them, though without any resolution. Mark would remain silently pre-occupied with the fight, his rage and his anxiety. Joanna, however, appeared able to dismiss the intensity of their disagreement. She had many individual friends from work and the neighborhood. He had only one friend, whom he saw infrequently. Even when the couple would attempt a compromise, Mark felt that Joanna's interest and effort were not enough and Joanna felt his demands were insatiable.

The couples' therapist they were seeing attempted a psychoeducational/CBT approach to negotiating their differences. After a year, that treatment ended without much change. The second couples' therapist focused on issues of attachment. Mark had a pre-occupied attachment with intense anxiety which could only be quelled with contact from Joanna. Joanna had an avoidant attachment where she wanted less contact, less emotional involvement and felt Mark to be intrusive into her space. Mark would remain intensely pre-occupied with the lack of intimacy and would go through periods of distrust, attempting to check up on her by reading her emails. Joanna, however, was able to gain psychological distance from the conflict and utilized her many affiliative relationships to reduce her distress and meet her intimacy needs. They differed in their perceptions of what constituted intimacy and were fairly inflexible and resistant to change. Yet when Mark eventually would withdraw, become depressed and resolve to leave, Joanna would make a significant effort to meet his demands for a short time. At some point, Joanna would become psychologically depleted, unable to sustain the effort, and withdraw. The cycle would then repeat with Mark silently pre-occupied and then demanding. When Joanna would accommodate, Mark would be angry that he had to insist.

Joanna felt loved by her parents. Nonetheless, she described them as fairly strict, no-nonsense, unemotional, 'suck-it-up' individuals, attitudes they conveyed to their children. Mark described his mother as narcissistic and his father as ineffectual. In order to keep the connection, he became anxious and hypervigilant to their emotional states. This second couples' therapist made modest progress in helping each recognize the differences in their relational styles and emotionality, how it developed and unfolded in their interactions. Each developed some empathy for the other.

One interesting aspect to each of their styles was that Mark would attempt to directly enlist the help of the couples' therapist privately, articulating his dissatisfaction, but often would not confront Joanna, hoping that the therapist would do so. Joanna and Mark had different abilities for recognizing their own desire for care and for being able to ask when it was needed. Mark's expectation to have the therapist articulate his needs to Joanna rather than asking directly for himself highlights the differences in couples' expectations about what others should 'know'.

Intimate couples feel free to disclose parts of themselves that they would not disclose to others, both positive and negative emotions. In an interesting study of newlyweds over a two-year period with daily diary recordings, attachment was linked to the quality of interactions and conflict (Feeney, Noller, & Callan, 1994). When husbands were comfortable with closeness and intimacy, they were more disclosing, more involved and more satisfied in the relationship. In contrast, when wives had high attachment anxiety, they were more dissatisfied and experienced conflicts as more coercive and distressing. When anxiety and avoidance levels are high, there is less likely to be trust and support which will likely result in poor conflict management, lack of intimacy and more relationship dissatisfaction (Khalifian & Barry, 2016).

Interest in obtaining care and ability to seek it when needed

Desiring care and having the ability to seek it is likely to be an innate predisposition as it enhances survival. One has to trust that others are available for sensitive and responsive care. Research suggests that when both preschool and school age children are securely attached, they have positive representations of their mothers as available responsive and comforting. They are comfortable in seeking care. As secure adolescents and adults begin new relationships, they expect and trust that others accept them, will provide care if they need it and that this will contribute to intimacy (Cassidy, 2001). Children with avoidant attachments have mothers who are often uncomfortable with close bodily contact. These children have difficulty seeking care. In the Strange Situation, these children when separated from their primary caregiver used 'diversionary activity' to deal with the separation, focusing on the toys, rather than the separation. They appear not to be bothered by the separation, but autonomic indicators indicate an increase in heart rate, rather than a decrease which usually accompanies genuine play (Spangler & Grossman, 1993). These children were found to more likely make eye-contact when they were not distressed. They lack representations of their mothers as supportive. As their mothers have modeled, they too deny the importance of the primary relationship. Adults with avoidant attachments have trouble seeking care.

Clinical vignette: 2

Lucinda, a young adult, lived with her parents after college, although finances were such that this was not a necessity. However, she rarely ate with her family and resented having to socialize with them. She described her mother as having 'sharp edges' and her father as being warmer, but more invested in his work than in his family. Lucinda said that she hated to be touched by her family members but enjoyed physical touch by her friends. However, most of her friends were online and there were few she actually met in person. She wished for a partner, but overtures of intimacy were met with disdain.

When her mother was dying, Lucinda expressed impatience for it to occur. During her mother's decline, she rejected bids to spend time with her mother. When her mother died, she expressed resentment at funeral attendance, felt imposed upon when having to plan the rituals of the funeral with her family, and did not find comfort when relatives visited and mourned. Around the same time, her usually pristine attention to appearance deteriorated and she appeared disheveled. The therapeutic relationship mirrored her other relationships. She was overtly rejecting of its significance, frequently found fault with the therapist for not providing adequate care and support, but never missed a session over a number of years.

When mothers are inconsistent and at the same time overly intrusive, children become hypervigilant. These children with insecure ambivalent attachment are not calmed by a reunification after a separation. There is an exaggerated negative emotion which tends to become chronic. During adulthood, this hyperactivation takes the form of a pre-occupying desire for intense closeness. Although initially this might give rise to an acceptable form of attention and interest in others, in the long term it leads to feeling threatened when a partner strives for autonomy and personal growth. The earlier example of Mark provides an illustration.

With insecure disorganized attachment, the baby and child seek care from someone who frightens them. Mental representations of mothers as hostile, violent and incoherent are prevalent, and this interferes with intimacy with another as there is little trust that the relationship can be counted on.

Clinical vignette: 3

Mira, a woman in her mid-30s, provides an example. Although she was professionally successful and physically quite attractive, most of her romantic involvements were limited to one-night stands. Memories of her mother included the horrible awareness that her mother was willing to sell Mira for sex when she was barely an adolescent in order to obtain drugs. Although the patient stated that she desired an intimate connection, she was frightened and distrustful of seemingly genuine attempts by others in that direction. She expressed ambivalence about desire to be cared for and loved. She involved herself with men who enjoyed bondage and occasionally found herself engaging in sadistic acts as well. Periods of her dissociation were confusing to the partner who remained interested as she vacillated between clinging and avoidant presentations.

Capacity to give care when needed

The ability to recognize that someone needs care and to be sensitive to the kind of care needed and then able to provide it fosters an intimate connection (Cassidy, 2001). Caregiving includes emotional and instrumental support; it enhances psychological wellbeing by reducing the partner's distress and supporting their personal growth by providing a secure base. One's attachment experiences influence their expectations for the social support that they expect to receive. Having received appropriate care, children develop an orientation that others can be relied upon for support. The components of caregiving that have been most researched are sensitivity and responsiveness.

Sensitivity is whether one can detect distress and match the kind and amount of support that someone needs and wants. Secure children as young as 4 are able to recognize distress in another (Cassidy, 2001). Secure adults are more likely than insecure ones to offer care and sensitive support to their partners (Feeney, 1996). Insecure adults sometimes seem unaware that their partners need support or offer insensitive support. Research suggests that individuals seem to glean the most psychological benefit from support when they are not consciously aware that they are receiving the support (Bolger & Amarel, 2007).

Responsiveness to the awareness of needed care is also an important aspect of intimacy. A study with married couples found secure attachment is associated with beneficial caregiving and satisfaction in the marriage (Feeney, 1996). Those with secure attachments are comfortable with intimacy and more readily trust. Those pre-occupied and fearful depend upon others for self-worth and worry about their relationships. Secure individuals give more responsive and less compulsive care. Avoidant individuals are less sensitive and give lower levels of responsive care. Pre-occupied and fearful individuals give more than is needed or wanted. Levels of sensitivity and responsiveness are also state dependent, varying upon the individual's mood (Iida, Seidman, Shrout, Fujita, & Bolger, 2008).

Clinical vignette: 4

John and Jane, newly married a year ago, had an argument in the morning before John left for work. If both had been securely attached, their anger at each other would likely dissipate over the day; they might soul search for their contributions and consider how the other might need the rupture repaired. There would be discussion either during the day or that evening and having both resolved to communicate needs more directly, they might have enjoyed an intimate evening. Because of trust in the permanence of the relationship and openness to feedback, neither would feel overwhelming anxiety to immediately and throughout the day attempt to resolve the problem. They would consider whether a response would be needed before the day's end. However, this was not the case for this couple.

John continued to process the argument on his way to work. He could not concentrate at work. During his lunch hour, he bought some roses and then surprised Jane with the flowers. Jane took the flowers and verbally thanked him, but John felt her response was not heart-felt especially because she did not give him a hug. He went back to work and became increasingly angry at her lack of appreciation and the lack of physical contact. Jane was also angry. She viewed his returning home with flowers as a thinly veiled distrust of her, experiencing the surprise as an intrusion in her day. Neither John nor Jane was able to respond appropriately to the other. Instead, each projected their own anxiety and distrust upon the other. Neither had an empathic stance. Although at a conscious level, John felt he was making attempts to repair the rupture, he did so without considering how his gesture might be perceived. Jane, on the other hand, behaved like most insecure individuals who are less likely to perceive such gestures as supportive (Pietromonaco & Beck, 2015). Were the two partners securely attached, one would have provided appropriate care and the other accepted it with grace.

Capacity to be at ease with the autonomous self

Autonomy is important to intimacy because it allows one to be close without fears of engulfment. The attachment system interacts with the exploratory system to foster a secure attachment. A secure base is necessary for exploration because the child needs to feel that the secure base is available if there is danger. Several longitudinal studies (Cassidy & Main, 1984; Cassidy, 2001) have supported the link between secure attachment and autonomy in children. Those who are insecure are less likely to explore and engage in autonomous play.

Feeney and Thrush (2010) have articulated three aspects of a secure base in adult relationships. First, partners need to feel that the other is available in case they need support. Second, when they do need support, the support should not interfere with exploration. Third, encouragement of exploration needs to be communicated. The secure base allows for a 'dependency paradox'. When individuals are comfortable having their partner depend upon them, their partners are abler to pursue and achieve their own goals (Feeney, 2015; Feeney, Van Vleet, & Jakubiak, 2015). The secure base, even in adulthood, encourages exploration and personal growth. Those with insecure attachment anxiety have difficulty allowing for such dependence if they anticipate that this will further separate them from their partner, as is suggested by this next case.

Clinical vignette: 5

Jake and Joan had been married for 15 years. Joan had been the primary breadwinner for the family. After their child was born two years into their marriage, they decided that Joan had more earning potential so Jake should remain home with the child until he began school. Both described feeling secure with each other and happy in their relationship. Jake enjoyed being a father and accepted the role reversal, although he had few supports in the community. Joan made enormous leaps in her career.

However, Joan and Jake gradually began to communicate less, enjoy fewer intimate moments and feel increasingly isolated from each other. Jake made some effort to return to work after their son was in fifth grade but Joan's hectic work schedule made it difficult for her to share in child care responsibilities. She encouraged Jake to remain home for another six months. Joan, however, made no effort to change her work schedule. Jake felt frustrated, trapped, increasingly depressed and distant. Joan too felt that she had lost the support of her husband and began to experience anxieties and doubt about pursuing further career goals.

Jake began therapy after another two years, in the depths of a depressive episode. Family work with them enabled Jake to experience Joan as a secure base to pursue a career. Joan too had to deal with her fears of losing Jake's support and losing Jake's attentions to a new career.

In this example, while both appeared to have secure attachments as a foundation, circumstances seemed to lead to the deterioration of their secure and intimate relationship. A number of quantitative studies (see Feeney, 2016 for a review of this literature) have examined the stability of adult romantic attachments over various time intervals. No matter what the time interval, it appears that approximately one-fourth of the participants change attachment type over time. Environmental circumstances such as loss can affect attachment style. Likely though, early adverse events may make some individuals more prone to this.

Capacity to negotiate

In close relationships, although there might be similar styles, there will never be a complete synchrony as shared events may activate different responses. Thus, for intimacy to be maintained, the ability to negotiate with each other is paramount. Such skills of negotiation originate during the last stage of early attachment when mother and child mutually work out the optimal distance between them so that the child can explore within a secure base while mother can tend to her own needs. The child is able to experience and express negative emotions and frustrations, and the mother is able to accomplish tasks that may involve other people or things. Both are able to successfully negotiate so that each will get some of their needs met. In a study of romantic couples (Feeney, 1994), secure individuals were found to have better ability to negotiate and to view it as mutual compared to insecure individuals. Related to this is the ability to confront conflict without being psychologically overwhelmed and then to be responsive to the other's demands. As expected, those with avoidant attachment styles overestimated their partner's negative emotions and underestimated their partner's appropriate responsiveness. They were more likely to be hostile and defensive in the discussion (Beck, Pietromonaco, DeVito, Powers, & Boyle, 2014; Overall, Fletcher, Simpson, & Fillo, 2015).

Conclusion

Attachment bonds and intimacy are intricately woven into neurobiological foundations. Early attachment experiences with primary caregivers impact the capacity to develop and maintain meaningful relationships in adulthood. Indeed, attachment preferences influence nearly all features of intimacy. Attachment styles differentially affect requirements of intimate relationships. Attachment preferences determine preferred affect regulation strategies and bias perceptions of intimate behavior by impacting attention and memory of intimate moments and conflictual interactions. Attachment styles influence the capacity to ask for and receive support in times of distress, to encourage growth in a partner and negotiate differences in distress tolerance, and comfort and personal growth desired.

Notes

1 In this contribution, we frequently refer to the primary attachment figure as maternal as most primary attachments are to the biological mother. However, the primary attachment bond can be a father or other male, relative or adoptive parent.
2 The infant and child's attachment system utilizes a multitude of behaviors to achieve the security needed. For example, walking and crawling may have the same functional equivalency within this motivational system, differing depending upon development (Sroufe & Waters, 1977). At a later point in development, the child can call up an image of the mother and experience a felt security which serves a similar function to the direct contact needed when younger. Also, the same behavior may serve multiple systems; when a child approaches the mother it may be for security and proximity needs, but it also could a desire to play, part of the sociability behavioral system (Cassidy, 2016).
3 Multiple attachments do develop over the first year with father, siblings and other family serving as competent caregivers and providers of security (Howes & Spieker, 2016). An 'attachment hierarchy' usually exists and broadens over the lifespan. Cassidy (2016) suggests that there is a 'reciprocal hierarchical bonding' where a child matches their attachment hierarchy to those attachment priorities in caregiving of others around them. This process increases the chances of survival if the child recognizes who is most bonded to them.
4 However, life events and the emergence of new and important relationships may modify internalized working models of attachment bonds throughout the lifespan (Feeney, 2016).
5 See Brabender and Fallon (2013) for a review.
6 In an analysis of 64 research studies published after these meta-analyses, parent caregiving also was found to be correlated with adult attachment (Jones, Cassidy and Shaver, 2015).
7 Within homogeneous environments and populations, heritability is higher than when there is greater heterogeneity (Bakersmans-Kranenburg & Van Ijzendoorn, 2016). This suggests that children might differ in their receptivity to parents' consistency and bids for a physical and emotional relationship (Belsky, 1997).
8 For pregnant women (and thereafter) there is an increasing level of estrogen which triggers an increase in oxytocin receptors in the forebrain. In rats, injecting oxytocin increases maternal behavior and blocking it decreases maternal behavior.
9 The empirical conceptualization of attachment has changed from the 'style' approach which was begun by Bowlby and Ainsworth and the dimensional approach which is currently the more favored approach. The dimensional approach uses two orthogonal dimensions – anxiety and avoidance (Feeney, 2016). Those low in both are considered to have secure attachments. Individuals high in anxiety and low in avoidance are considered pre-occupied (anxious ambivalent). Those high in avoidance and low in anxiety are referred to as dismissing. Those high in both anxiety and avoidance are categorized as fearful (Fraley, 2010).

Chapter 3

Intimacy and its vicissitudes in adolescence

David Pauley

I begin this chapter on adolescent intimacy with a paradox, one echoed in the following diaphanous stanzas from Arthur Rimbaud's poem, "Romance", – written when the poet was 17, in 1870 – yet still fresh, as descriptive of the Snapchat generation as it is of each of the successive cohorts of youths who have encountered it (and grown older) in the intervening decades:

> When you are seventeen you aren't really serious.
> – One fine evening, you've had enough of beer and lemonade,
> And the rowdy cafes with their dazzling lights!
> – You go walking beneath the green lime trees of the promenade.
> The lime trees smell good on fine evenings in June!
> The air is so soft sometimes, you close your eyelids;
> The wind, full of sounds, – the town's not far away –
> Carries odors of vines, and odors of beer. (pp. 99–100)

Rimbaud's poem conjures up the impress of adolescent longing in ways that few other literary works manage to do, much less those of so diminutive a size (just 285 words in Bernard's translation) or composed by so youthful a poet. In achieving this susurrated alchemy, "Romance" also points toward a dilemma that many of us today face as we attempt to make sense of those same epochal yearnings: the dreamy, irreducible *sensory* nature of so much of adolescent experience, and its preternaturally stubborn resistance to verbal translation.

This paradox – on display as I embark on the current discussion – also figures in the helplessness that grips many parents as they attempt to weave a coherent narrative out of the often bewildering, contradictory postures of the teenagers in their lives. It also figures as well in the perhaps counterphobic comprehensiveness of efforts by professional psychotherapists to account for those same tendencies scientifically – from Peter Blos's classic (in many ways now woefully outdated) psychoanalytic studies *On Adolescence* (1968) and *The Adolescent Passage* (1979), to Daniel Siegel's more mass market-oriented, neurobiologically inflected and current *Brainstorm: The Power and Purpose of the Teenage Brain* (2015). Whatever the merits of such books, these types of efforts always carry about them a whiff of formaldehyde, a sense that adolescent motivations are, if not exactly pathological, then at the very least a puzzling sub-species of experience whose taxonomy can be catalogued by sober-minded adults – butterflies on a board – while eliding the sensory evidence obvious to most any poet (or teenager): the purpose of butterflies is *flight*.

Still, as adolescents arrive with their parents in increasing numbers in psychotherapists' offices, wracked with worries, large or small, it seems prudent to continue trying to trace the well-springs that feed them and occasionally drive them to distraction, well-springs we adults might once have known viscerally, but that are now (to invert the apostle's metaphor) glimpsed only 'through a glass darkly'. The scientific voice, with its probing questions and soothing generalities, definitely has a place in such discussions[1] but also has some not inconsiderable limitations that I will explore in the pages that follow. These limitations, common as well to the broader, ever-shifting cultural narrative of adolescence from which those medicalized confections spring, turn on questions of intimacy, those sensual-existential vibrations that ripple through the youthful subject of Rimbaud's poem, embodied a few lines later in the form of a young girl in her "little ankle boots" strolling the same walkway under the watchful eye of her father. A certain narrow reading of "Romance", or a similar gloss on the psychoanalytic literature of adolescence, might conclude that the intimacy yearned for here is that of a love affair, or at least that of a 'hookup,' yet Rimbaud's poem, which follows the young man through the first thunderclap of attraction and later intense epistolary pursuit of his beloved, arrives at a surprising ending which belies such facile interpretations:

> – Then your adored one, one evening, condescends to write to you . . . !
> That evening, – you go back again to the dazzling cafes,
> You ask for beer or for lemonade . . .
> – You are not really serious when you are seventeen
> And there are green lime trees on the promenade . . . (pp. 99–100)

This unforeseen, bracingly adolescent pivot provoked sighs of appreciation from my high school French teacher when she recited this poem for my 10th grade class in the early 1980s[2] but was undoubtedly received by my teenage self, and by a great many of my peers at that juncture, with eye-rolling, even stupefaction ("The girl finally wrote him back and he got rid of her? What's the point?").

Elucidating that 'point', trying to situate it within the broader cultural conversation on adolescence – which exists in the perspective-skewing, sideview-mirror recollections of parents and psychotherapists, and gets imprinted afresh each day on the kinetic, Rorschach-like surfaces of teenage bodies – is the goal of this chapter.

The body as map and mirror

The first proposition I will take up – it hovers lightly in the background of Rimbaud's poem, but echoes like a hammer in Blos's text and also (if a bit more artfully) in Siegel's more heterodox, mass-market interpretation – holds that such intimate longings, like the pubertal changes that herald their onset, are primarily physiological events, bound up in the cascading instinctual and neurobiological transformations of the teenage years. For Blos, as for most psychoanalytic 'drive theorists' going back to Freud, this framing was axiomatic. The seething libidinal and aggressive energies of infancy, banked into serviceable fires during the elementary school years, overtake their fragile enclosures with the arrival of puberty, laying waste to the flimsy defensive adaptations of that earlier period, requiring a wholesale renovation and expansion of the ego and all but guaranteeing chaotic flare-ups in teenagers' interpersonal behavior (pitched rebellion against chafing parental strictures; bodily experimentation of all stripes, including that of a symptomatic flavor) en route to biologically pre-determined end-points. For Blos and many analysts of his era (e.g. Anna Freud, 1965; Erikson, 1985), those end-points in the best case included procreative heterosexual couple-hood and the assumption of normative gender roles that would not only ensure the propagation of the species but the preservation of a kind of reassuring, blue-chip bodily and familial aesthetic (Blos, 1968). This outcome, whose stodginess at one moment may have been derided by teenagers (or feared – the girl's father in Rimbaud's poem sports a "terrifying stiff collar"), is in the end accepted and even embraced as form-fitting and *natural* as they plunge through the churning cataracts into adulthood.

Seigel's text, reflective of the more varied relational menu awaiting today's youth, treads lightly on questions of normative gender expectations (gay desire makes a belated but not unwelcome appearance, though trans experience, to say nothing of the corrosive impact of sexism or racism, are not touched on),[3] but still blurs the boundary between the biological and social transformations of the teenage years. Its author is on solid ground as he recaps findings of neurobiology, phenomena now readily observable through PET scans and other technological lenses. Examples of this include the suggestive 'pruning' and gradual insulation of neural connections in the adolescent brain, or the context-specific drench of dopamine that serves to reward adolescent risk-taking, and may also explain many teenagers' twitching aversion to (comparatively unrewarded) periods of quiescence, at least until a more enduring equilibrium is established. Such potent but creeping structural changes in the makeup of the nervous system – beyond the power of earlier generations of researchers to glimpse – is accompanied in "Brainstorm" by a smattering of findings from cognitive science that is similarly evocative. The most widely applicable of these is Seigel's description of the comparatively late arrival of so-called 'gist thinking' in the teenage years, a cognitive leap whose earlier absence informs the seemingly endless, half-baked ways in which adolescents arrive at decisions that lack the essential leavening of common sense. This tendency was on display in my office recently in dramatic fashion as a 15-year-old defended her desire to engage with her boyfriend in 'urban exploration' – scaling bridges and half-built skyscrapers in the quest for thrills and artistically composed selfies. Not even the several recent death plunges covered in the press were enough to dissuade the young woman from this pursuit; rather than being received in a cautionary spirit (*this could happen to you!*) – a 'gist' that would be readily grasped by many slightly older persons – the young woman saw the senseless deaths as statistical support for relative safety of the undertaking (a handful of incidents in a city of 8 million over many months – *why worry?*). Most therapists would be apt to see this kind of blinkered rationalization as intrinsically pathological (evidence of a barely contained suicidal impulse, for example, or stemming from the young woman's unhealthy obeisance to her boyfriend's wishes), but Seigel's text makes clear that such head-scratching (occasionally tragic) mis-readings may also arise from a transient, age-specific glitch in the brain's perceptual sub-routines – one that, he observes, argues for the continued close monitoring of teenagers by adults.

The one major area where Seigel veers into epistemologically dicey territory, is, ironically, the very place his text seems to regard as securely charted ground, as illustrated in the following passage from an early, theme-setting chapter, "The Essence of Adolescence":

> Two things happen universally in our human adolescence. One is that as puberty hits we begin to experience changes in the body and changes in our emotions. The second is that we push away from our parents, hanging out with our peers more and trying to do things in new ways.
>
> (p. 25)

While the first of these two claims is far from controversial – adolescents across cultures do indeed, by definition, go through profound physiological and emotional changes that start at puberty and don't settle down until the early to mid-20s – Seigel's second observation, about the pushing away from parents and hanging out with peers, is (as he must surely know) anything but universal. A wealth of historical and anthropological data point one in the opposite direction: 'separation-individuation,'[4] the dominant developmental narrative of adolescent experience in Western countries like the present-day United States (and the one to which his account most closely hews), is very much a cultural and historical construct – one that, notwithstanding Seigel's universalist claims, may very possibly be receding at the present moment, morphing, under our noses, into different, if not yet fully hatched, new patterns (see, for example, Twenge & Park, 2017).

Individuation: the quest for intimacy and its perils

One can marshal data in support of such a (perhaps controversial) contention in all kinds of ways, the most obvious of which – for a chapter like this in the tradition of psychoanalytic writing – would be to look at the relevant literature and then perhaps fold in some case material to illustrate the points in question. While I will certainly do some of that in the pages that follow, I will depart from that convention, for a while least, to have a look at this topic on a more distinctly personal level, as it has developed over the past two generations in my family and is coalescing at the current moment in the rather different cultural and historical circumstances of my 10-year-old daughter's life. This type of personal narrative-making, which has a precedent in certain corners of our field – the path-breaking (Menninger-trained) family systems therapist Murray Bowen is one notable early proponent – remains far from the norm in psychoanalytic discourse, but, one hopes, may become increasingly widespread as clinicians plumb the recesses of their personal histories (extensively mapped in their training analyses) by way of providing greater nuance and specificity to our theories (Bowen, 2004). On emotionally laden topics like adolescence, it should go without saying, those theoretical models never exist in a conceptual vacuum but always bear the imprint of the diverse places from which we come.

In many ways, my small-town, middle-class American childhood could be seen as unfolding according to the classic pattern of separation-individuation, as brought into the developmental discourse of adolescence by Blos and similar thinkers. My four elder brothers and I, born toward the end of the so-called 'baby boom' years (between 1955 and 1965), grew up in an environment of widespread material abundance, without the wrenching economic and global-historical shocks that had marked the coming of age of our parents and grandparents. After some quite dramatic chapters of upheaval between 1970 and 1988 when the bulk of us were in the adolescent maelstrom – 'hippie'-like long hair, psychedelic drugs, rock music and an often militant rejection of authority were the order of the day – we plunged into the capillary-like system of highways criss-crossing our home county and took up residence in distant parts of the country, ranging from hundreds to thousands of miles from the family nest. My parents, both conventional middle class college grads, without ever necessarily formulating the thought as such, had always looked to school to be the engine that helped chaperone their five sons into maturity, but were on the whole – like more than a few parents of their generation – greatly disappointed in this. Concrete proof of this disenchantment persisted, for many years, in a locked file cabinet with their financial papers: five neatly tallied custodial savings account passbooks, flush with funds amassed diligently over many years and earmarked for our future college tuition that only two of us ended up using.

My father, the older of my parents by eight years and a proud member of what came much later to be called the 'greatest generation', took all of this especially hard. The low point for him came in the mid-1970s and was embodied in the person of my brother Kevin, a flame-headed imp in the middle of the pack, who went from being a fairly benign presence – a bit of a cut-up, the butt of (mostly) good-natured joshing – to a frightening, almost unrecognizably feral creature. Wholly ungovernable for a time, Kevin found himself drawn to high school dropouts and all manner of 'low-lifes' (his word) whom he followed – or, more likely, *led* – with seeming relish, into pursuits unthinkable by our straight-laced elders: extensive drug experimentation and dealing, petty crimes ranging from vandalism to house-breaking, sexual escapades hinted at but never, to me at least, enumerated. He sported a crude, homemade tattoo memorializing some of these, a source of pride that – in the way of such things – became faintly embarrassing to him in later life.

Perhaps unsurprisingly, though Kevin drifted through his teenage years without ever acquiring a diploma (or any other badge of academic distinction), he also became acquainted with other institutions that shaped his adulthood, from juvenile detention centers and psychiatric wards to a white-pillared military academy – our World War II veteran father's last, desperate effort at keeping his third-born son from hitting the shoals. Kevin acceded to that placement, proffered as an alternative to more time in 'juvie', with surprising equanimity, bearing his neck even for the required haircut, but eyed the manicured campus when we accompanied him there – its stables, rifle range and athletic fields – with a bemused, even ironic detachment (he absconded within weeks of arriving).

Kevin's travails in adolescence, higher-octane versions of the concussions that rocked each of our lives to varying degrees in those years, existed in a realm beyond the powers of my parents, or indeed any of us, to conceptualize verbally. If pressed at the time to speak about whatever dark forces were animating his actions, I doubt sincerely he could have done so, so much was he enmeshed in the sensory experience of them. Kevin very likely would have mouthed the word 'freedom' – that familiar rallying cry of teenagers, and one that in my family, as in many others, invited the inevitable, often pointless rejoinder ("if freedom is what you want, then why not buckle down and study and do what's necessary to get ahead in life?"). Kevin's yearning for liberty was, unfortunately, never the rational argument that my parents might have hoped for, but viewed from the vantage point of the present appears more like the manic writhing of a colt, thrashing its way through floodwaters toward some dimly scented, perhaps unreachable patch of ground.

My parents' narrative of Kevin's adolescent crisis, as cobbled together then and years afterward, leaned heavily on blame, and increasingly, self-blame. My father supposed that if only they had gotten him involved sooner in a more highly structured school environment (the military academy, or perhaps the up-market prep school that I attended years later), they might have disrupted his morbid involvement with his friends, a shift that could have made all the difference. My mother, less sanguine about such external changes (she grasped intuitively that the problem resided *within* Kevin, not just in his peer group or his school), wondered for years about various emotional factors extending back well into childhood that, if somehow untangled, might have set him on a smoother path: my father's at times blazing temper; the perhaps less innocent than previously thought joshing that shadowed Kevin throughout his childhood; the inevitable leaching away of focus and patience for his specific needs as my parents grappled with the clamorous demands of four other growing sons (including me, the late-arriving baby). I added to my mother's litany of self-reproaches for a time in my early 20s by sharing my own impressions of her flaws, pieced together in my first extended experience of psychotherapy – an almost irresistible (if sadistic) form of score-settling, with the adolescent Kevin as proxy for my own complaints about childhood.

As I have grown older in tandem with the adult Kevin – his adolescence thankfully did not end in tragedy, though the patterns he established there, drug abuse in particular, led to a significantly fore-shortened life (he died of an overdose at age 49) – I have become less certain about those blaming narratives, morality tales that seek to give one an illusion of agency within tectonic shiftings vaster and more impersonal than any individual actor. Viewed from the distant promontory of the present, where I am not only the anxious parent of a soon-to-be teen, but a therapist with a quarter-century's worth of contact with teenagers and their (often equally anxious) parents, I am compelled to conclude that Kevin's adolescence, for whatever ways in which it fits seamlessly into a psychoanalytic narrative of teenage pathology of the sort that Blos or Anna Freud might have penned – a germ of neglect, embryonic since toddlerhood, bursting from its chrysalis as a malignant rebellion with the onset of puberty – is in certain ways ill-served by that kind of arm-chair tautology, which pays too little heed to the ways in which wider cultural factors were also interlaced with his problems. Parsing out those cultural factors – beliefs and lived practices about selfhood, parenthood, child-rearing and family – can never lead one to the certainties of a PET scan read-out, but can, if one allows, perhaps engender a healthy skepticism about some of the seeming givens in our cultural discourse about adolescence, givens that, like the pieties at the heart of any folklore, can enhance one's appreciation for the unique teenagers in one's life, but also blind one to other, generative ways of grasping our collective struggle.

'Me' vs. 'we': culture as adolescent framework and buffer

My first clue that the separation-individuation/pushing away from parents story that both Blos and Daniel Seigel subscribe to as biologically driven was less than a universal experience came in my first job after graduate school, at a child guidance clinic located on a bustling crossroads in Flushing, Queens. At the Trude Weishaupt Clinic, we worked with families and children from across the globe, many of them recent immigrants; a significant part of our efforts with them focused on mediating the at times overwhelming conflicts that ensued as they contended with the very different norms and expectations of their adopted country as applied to the children and adolescents in their lives. The most bewildering aspect of this cultural disconnect for many of those families, and one that has been explored extensively in the literature (Mishne, 2002; Akhtar & Kramer, 1998), turned on the question of adolescent separation-individuation, and, in particular, the role assigned to parents in that process. Far from normative, the dominant American model of parenting adolescents – the ever-anxious, *laissez-faire* attitude that teenagers seemed to view, along with fast food and overpriced sneakers, as something of a birthright – for these parents appeared just as often as a threatening, almost comical abdication of parental authority. Time and again my co-workers and I ran interference on these kinds of questions, as the parents we worked with struggled to find some way to reconcile themselves to their relative wholly unfamiliar powerlessness to shape the choices of their 'separating, individuating' sons and daughters, and the seeming indifference, even hostility, of American institutions (from schools to mental health clinics to child welfare authorities) to ally with them in re-establishing an effective chain of command. As I worked with such families clinically and shared their struggles, it became increasingly clear to me that the adolescent crisis that is seen as such a given in our culture is very far from the norm in other parts of the world. Rather than something immutable, the expression of an endogenous, even Darwinian imperative (Siegel, 2015, p. 75), this type of transitory identity crisis and turning away from parental authority in favor of the peer group were starting to look much more like a culture bound syndrome, a kind of phase-specific madness we Americans and the wider culture we embody require of our youth as a rite of passage from the intimacy of childhood into the wholly different forms of intimate relationships characteristic of maturity.

Along with my work in that polyglot clinical community, my interest in the cultural cross-currents that shape life stages like adolescence gathered steam around the same time as I started that job, with my growing immersion in the extended family of my husband, a New Delhi-born Punjabi whose relatives, spread over two continents, were nonetheless still an important presence in his life. The difference in our cultural backgrounds created some challenges at the outset (coming out as gay was far from common in the milieu in which he grew up), but, once he introduced me to his relatives, did not negate their culturally inflected obligation, not only to be welcoming to me as a person, but to try to find a method of weaving me into their extended family tapestry in ways that corresponded to familiar roles (in my case, as a son-in-law, brother-in-law and uncle). One would perhaps expect the same kind of transition to unfold in my own family, and, to an extent, it did; my husband came in time to forge significant bonds with my relatives in ways that were little different than they might have been had we been in a traditional, heterosexual marriage, a fact which in itself speaks to the malleability of family culture: neither my churchgoing grandparents nor the piously Hindu elders in my husband's family would have found any support or even a normative frame of reference for welcoming LBGTQ grandchildren and their partners into their midst.

Despite a similar embrace from each family, however, the culture of family life into which I entered with his relatives (and have lived within for 25 years) was starkly different than the one I had grown up within, and this difference was especially pronounced as applied to care of the children and teenagers in the mix. The psychoanalyst Alan Roland, a longstanding observer of cultural differences between North Americans and South Asians as they enact the rituals of family life, has coined the term 'we self' to evoke this different developmental trajectory. Rather than the dominant 'me self' model of maturation common in Western societies – a sort of colonial enmeshment between the generations that comes to an abrupt, often stormy end with the Declaration of Independent Selfhood that accompanies the teenage years – Roland frames South Asian families as occupying a kind of loose and mutually reinforcing confederation of interests across generations that goes through an evolution with the onset of puberty, but never a definitive breach.

This 'we self'/'me self' distinction seemed most readily and viscerally graspable to me as I contended with the contrasting views that our two families had on the dominant role that my partner and I played vis-à-vis the next generation (until years later when we had our own child), that of uncle. My brothers and sisters-in-law on the 'American'[5] side of the family certainly hoped for a greater degree of warmth and connection from us as uncles than the desultory bond we had experienced with our own parents' siblings in childhood, yet we all understood instinctively that our involvement carried with it a culturally sanctioned set of boundaries, a deference to their role as parents and central attachment figures that, seen from afar, might very easily be characterized as a species of disinterest. Practically speaking, this meant that we were free to enjoy our nieces and nephews, products of my brothers' individuated/separated households, but would never have presumed (or been expected) to take on a quasi-parental role with them – to change diapers or soothe them to sleep, advise them or their parents meaningfully about the choices in their lives, or take on a sustained material or affective role in their care. This sort of smiling but arms-length avuncular relationship, with its pronounced deference to parents as the nucleus of children's lives, also later characterized the relationships between our daughter and her 'American' uncles, aunts and cousins, and was thus something created and actively reproduced by that 'American' family, *including us*, as a system, not imposed from without.

On the 'Indian' side of the family, things could not have been more different. Long before I came into that family, my husband had played the role of doting, minutely involved uncle to his siblings' children, one whose opinions factored significantly into their parents' decisions about their care. When visiting, he would enjoy an intimacy with the children, including a *physical* intimacy – feeding, bathing, brushing teeth, cuddling, that was very much expected to not only support but temporarily *eclipse* that of the parents. That younger generation, in turn – especially our two nephews who grew up in the U.S. – enjoyed a relationship with him, and later with me, that was far more intimate and differentiated (i.e. direct – not just filtered through parental wishes) than any I experienced with the younger generation of our family until we had our own daughter years later.

The proof of this intimate bond was made manifest during our nephews' adolescence and young adulthood. Even as their relationships with their parents became occluded by some of the storminess one associates with typical forms of adolescent estrangement, they maintained their expected roles within the extended family – dutifully catering to the elders living nearby or visiting from India, while un-ambivalently, even joyfully playing the role of 'elder brother' (*bhaiya*) to younger cousins, all the while deriving support and relational sustenance, and a degree of respite from their parents, in the homes of uncles, aunts and elder cousins (including ours, where both nephews lived for varying periods of time in their late teens and 20s). Thus, even as they also forged important relationships with peers and negotiated the at times daunting thickets of American identity-making as evoked by Erickson – choices about peer groups, academic and career interests, romantic partners, moral values, fashion and musical taste, religious attitudes (all of which unfolded in the ambivalent shadow of parental expectation) – those two young men also enjoyed what one might think of as multiple 'conflict-free' realms of experience, safe ports within the extended family where identity continued to unfold according to predictable, socially gratifying patterns (Erikson, 1968).

My reading of the literature on cross-cultural psychoanalysis, taken in conjunction with direct observation of numerous other Indian and Pakistani families within and outside of the clinical realm over many years, makes clear that this kind of intimate evolution within extended families – not 'a breach, but an expansion' (to borrow another poet, Donne's (1611), famous phrase) – is far from uncommon, and may indeed still be a norm for much of that community both in the North American diaspora and on the subcontinent. That transgenerational interdependence – 'we self' – may reach a kind of crucial apogee in the adolescent years, but it makes its first appearance in the early months of life, a fact described most extensively by anthropologist Stanley Kurtz in a compelling chapter in a 1992 volume of analytically derived ethnography applied to child-rearing on the Indian subcontinent (Kurtz, 1992). Kurtz's book received some justified criticism from analytic writers such as Salman Akhtar, who questioned its repeated assertion to the effect that Indian mothers, while *physically* permissive in matters of nursing and co-sleeping with young children, display a striking lack of *emotional* responsiveness and warmly engaged mirroring of their children's self states as compared with their North American counterparts, an absence that – as Akhtar observes – flies in the face of even the most perfunctory observation of South Asian parents and children interacting in public places (Akhtar, 1997). While it is tempting to try to parse the reasons for this disjunction – a good bit of Kurtz's data seems to come from relatively impoverished rural *milieux*, much of it recorded in the literature in the 1960s or 1970s (see Minturn & Hitchcock, 1966; one wonders how empathic and mirroring American parents from remote parts of Appalachia might have appeared at that same moment, especially under the eye of a foreign observer) – Kurtz's broader point, as signaled in the title of his book, *All the Mothers Are One*, would seem to strongly bolster Roland's 'we self' formulation. That point, boiled down to its core, is that Indian mothers (and, I would add, fathers) nurture a relational system in which 'mothering' – and all of the attachment security, familiarity and intimacy it represents – is, from very early in life, diffused over a broader intergenerational family system, not constrained (as is the more common case in the West) within the exclusive purview of the parental couple, or in the sole person of the mother (Chodorow, 1978). Kurtz and Roland's observations about South Asian parenting and selfhood, which track very closely with my own observations of dynamics at play on the 'Indian' side of my bi-cultural extended family, have far-reaching implications not just for adolescent development, but for the whole analytic discourse on attachment, which takes the nuclear, mid-century Western family on whose experience it was based as normative and is replete with classist, heteronormative and sexist assumptions ripe for re-appraisal (Bowlby, 1969).

As far as adolescents are concerned, these cross-cultural conversations would seem to make clear that teenagers in different cultures do not start from the same 'average expectable environment' with regard to intimate attachments as they embark on the adolescent journey, but in fact enter puberty from strikingly different home bases from which they rove far and wide over the teenage years. Indian families like my husband's, to a degree that is uncommon in typical American nuclear families, often take pains to nurture an intimate middle ground (starting with the literal, bodily intimacy of multiple 'mothers' in childhood) that functions akin to a buffering Winnicottian 'transitional space' between the 'inside' world of the biological mother-child bond and the 'outside' world of peers, school and the wider community (Winnicott, 1953). A practical consequence of this fertile and enduring relational margin would seem to be that South Asian teenagers (and parents) enter the adolescent riptides with a far more varied and flexibly rooted support system in place, multiple nodes of intimate attachment across generations that function like so many steadying handholds as families together negotiate the at times dizzying transformation that adolescence brings.[6] Typical North American teenagers, in contrast, not unlike my brother Kevin decades ago, enter the teenage years without the same wide-ranging web of supports in place and rely instead, to a degree that is perhaps unusual in other parts of the world, on the unitary pillar of the parenting couple. That parent-teenager pillar, saturated from both ends with affective significance and intimacy based on early childhood experience, can ill withstand the many moltings – physiological, psychosexual, cultural, semiotic – that adolescence brings, and, as a result, often goes through a reactive constriction of intimacy that one might view, were it to crop up in a marriage such as a refusal to communicate meaningfully, a lack affection or interest, a hostility to reasonable behavioral accommodation as prelude to a divorce.

Economics, intimacy and separation: adolescence as an ambivalent exodus

How did things get to be this way? Our developmental theories tell us that this kind of temporary estrangement from family is normative, biologically driven, part and parcel of the neurological/intrapsychic remolding that adolescence brings. While this is often a useful narrative to have in one's pocket (what adolescent therapist hasn't at times endorsed the description of teenagers in her practice as unpredictable, authority-averse, hormonal hot messes?), this narrative, as I have sought to demonstrate, is in fact a scientific gloss on a predominantly Western (European, North American) bit of folklore, a folklore, moreover, that thinkers from the magisterial Phillipe Ariès (1962) to newer voices like the American historian Kent Baxter (2008) frame, ever more emphatically, as being of relatively recent vintage. While anything like a thorough overview of the historiography of childhood and adolescence would lead far afield of the current discussion, that literature in aggregate suggests that the Western notion of adolescence as a distinct developmental epoch[7] dates at the latest from the mid-19th century, as industrialization, more than any other factor, re-shaped the contours of family life across Europe and the U.S. Unlike agrarian societies, where having one's children close by was an economic necessity, not just on the farm but in the trades, with skills passed along from one generation to the next, the advent of industrialization exponentially intensified a demographic trend on the rise in Europe since the beginning of the colonial era that rewarded sallying forth – separating, individuating, planting one's flag on distant shores – as a means of making one's way in the world. That culture-defining economic imperative toward separation in the North American context did not lessen with the closing of the frontier symbolized by the linking up of the transcontinental railroads in the late 1860s, but in fact increased, as the industrial economy, making use of those same rail lines (and later, highways and aviation routes), molded a more fleet-footed and literate workforce ready to do its bidding and reap its material benefits.

Thus, at the very moment that industry was creating pools of economic opportunity open to youths willing to uproot themselves from distant parts of the country and the world, it was also fueling a parallel need for new generations of managers, inventors, scholars and teachers that together constituted another reservoir of opportunity for the era's teenagers, embodied in the educational system. This trend, as Baxter points out, is evident in the rapid construction of high schools in the latter half of the 19th century, where attendance was increasingly mandated by law, as well as in the ever-expanding, slowly democratizing realm of higher education. One sees abundant evidence of this relatively recent – at times vertiginous – formalizing of knowledge-transmission among generations of American youth in the recent history of a great many families. When my father entered college as a freshman on the eve of the Second World War, for example, only 4.6% of Americans held undergraduate degrees (Wilson, 2017). His tenure as a graduate business student in the decade after the war – paid for through the G.I. bill (and viewed with bemused skepticism by my self-tutored grandfather) – was a sufficient novelty at that juncture as to be irrelevant to my father's future career. He characteristically and perhaps not atypically never bothered to finish writing his MBA thesis. In the span of just a generation, however, undergraduate degrees – many of them involving relocating at a significant remove from the family home – have gone from being a status adornment held by a select few to a bare prerequisite for employment for a large segment of the population (not just the 33% who currently hold a bachelor's degree, but the far larger swath of the population that aspires and works ever more determinedly each year toward that distinction). Graduate degrees, similarly, have proliferated, becoming sought-after, often essential sources of 'cultural capital' among youth aspiring for a place in the professional, intellectual and managerial elites.

In working to set aside funds for our college education throughout the 1950s, 1960s and 1970s, therefore, my parents were not just as one might have supposed following the dictates of the gray-flannel world in which they had married, but were actively working to nudge us toward an enveloping structure – a transitional environment, if you will: new fields and pastures just over the next ridge – that would provide meaningful employment and a degree of economic security to each of us as we moved into adulthood. Unlike generations of parents in the pre-industrial era, however, their efforts, like those of the same cohort of parents in communities across the country, involved a tacit yet often quite wrenching bargain. To make good on those hopes, to bring those fertile uplands fully under the plow, their children would have to leave, to detach from the family geographically and emotionally and find their own paths, their own work and loves, and in time, their own, hermetically encapsulated experience of family, under other roofs. This rarely avowed but normative expectation of departure, evident in the alternatively saccharine or melancholy strains of so much of pop music and in the frenetic rituals of the teenage years from the politics of the peer group, sex and dating to college preparation, as much as any other factor of which I am aware, infuses the adolescent period at the present moment with its particular, culture-specific moodiness. Separation/individuation, less an intrapsychic epigenesis than an economic and cultural expectation, most certainly carries along with it a trove of pleasurable new possibilities, but also informs the piercing, at times overwhelming ambivalence that characterizes the adolescent passage, and not just for teenagers.

The journalist Jennifer Senior (2015), in her meticulously observed, expansive recent volume on parenting, *All Joy and No Fun*, describes with potent immediacy the toll that the adolescent passage takes on parents, as children (these days often less a biological inevitability than an active lifestyle choice) enter puberty and molt, transform and grow distant. Tapping away on their smartphones, gliding past social breakwaters into unseen vistas whose enticements and risks are all too easy to imagine, Senior's (and all of our) alternatively rebellious or taciturn teenagers are in fact obeying an exacting cultural itinerary beamed at them from every angle throughout the process of growing up: *Get away! Figure out what you want! Make your path in the world!* This enforced, lemming-like generational exodus, the defining feature of the Western teenage experience and the adult 'me self' that emerges from it, creates untold anxiety and even grief among parents as they grapple with the changes it wreaks, e.g. family nest heaving and splintering. Teens, either nonchalantly or dramatically, make choices at wide variance with parental expectations, and the upsurge in, at times, fearsome forms of symptomatic behavior from drug abuse to suicide attempts, accompanies the teenage years. All too often, however, as Senior's reporting and much daily clinical experience attests, parents – no less than therapists or the adults who pen our theories – frame these worrisome trends as encapsulated phenomena, unfolding solely within the opaque envelope of teenage bodies. In endorsing this common but obfuscating bit of scientifically sanctioned folklore, parents and therapists are deprived of a level of empowerment (and perhaps wisdom) that might come from seeing their own fingerprints, individually and collectively – their expectations and impossibly contradictory wishes ("Grow up!/Don't leave!"; "Find yourself!/ Do what I say!") – broadcast back, in relational semaphore, in their teenagers' restless peregrinations.

So it was, I believe, both in the stormy instance of separation-individuation epitomized decades ago in the experience of my brother Kevin, and, in not dissimilar ways, in the lyrical unfolding of the subject of Rimbaud's poem, and in the life of the poet himself, a century before. The symptomatic excesses of Kevin's passage through the adolescent maelstrom, so wrenching for all of us, for a time obscured his obvious, if lurching, outward trajectory. Kevin may have decisively rejected my parents' preferred *method* of separating from the nest and launching himself into adulthood, but, whatever his ambivalence, never contested their *goal*. In eschewing the outward shape of their dreams for him – turning away from formal education – he undoubtedly had a harder time of it than those of us whose adolescence hewed closer to the expected pathway, not in the least because of the resentment and hurt that his choices, and the brutal revision of those dreams, engendered. By his mid-20s, however, Kevin – mainly through informal interactions with his peer group – had indeed acquired an education of his own. While that less structured kind of learning never endowed him with the kind of academic badges that would have enabled him to join the ranks of the professions, or even to make sense of much of this current paper (he would certainly have gotten its gist, but would have found the language off-putting), he emerged into adulthood with a number of specialized skills – from laying tile to hanging doors or taping ups – whose value or humility depends entirely upon the relational context from which one observes them.

Rimbaud's poetic subject, based on the experience of the 17-year-old poet himself in the 1870s, comes into our awareness in a similar way, on a seemingly conventional path: a teenaged dreamer, out for a stroll, suddenly taken with the beauty surrounding him, and embodied most vividly in the fleeting form of the adolescent girl who captures his heart and, for a time, dominates his dreams. The poem's French title, "*Roman*", however, hints at an ambiguity, absent in Bernard's English translation, that is borne out in the poem's surprising trajectory. That word, which can, per Bernard, mean 'Romance', with all of the conventional narrative possibilities that it entails (the happily-ever-afters of love and marriage), can just as commonly be translated as "Novel", a broader and more sweeping narrative coming-into-being, and one that was beginning to unfold, increasingly at the time Rimbaud was writing, without the same pre-ordained end-points. As my high school French teacher might have put it, the 'romance' of the title is thus less about the girl as such than about the poet's relationship to his craft, including the words through which he woos her – as well as those later verses (the poem itself) in which he records the experience, and leads his chosen art form into unexpected and strikingly modern new directions.

Conclusion

Rimbaud, of course, was a rebel not just in art but in life, and for a time led a scandalous existence that (along with his growing renown) must have provoked bafflement and indignation in his piously authoritarian single mother. Homosexuality, rape, sadomasochism, drugs: Rimbaud's later poems – a catalogue of his experiences, and a foreshadowing of so many of the 'unspeakable' themes that have pre-occupied later generations of artists and teenagers – were all written before his 21st birthday, at which point he famously put down his pen and moved in a different direction. Far from returning, like a prodigal son, into the arms of his mother, the ex-poet roved even further from his native land, ultimately settling up shop as an itinerant coffee trader in Aden, Yemen, and in so doing, in ways that must have been all too clear to him, hewing closer than ever to the model of his scarcely remembered ship-captain father.

Would the poet have returned to writing had cancer not unexpectedly struck him down at the age of 38? Based on the scant historical evidence, this seems far from likely, though, reading his work, it is hard to shake one's desire for such a cinematic denouement: the mature poet, returning with fanfare to the embrace of the modern world that his youthful verses helped usher into being. A similar, no less wishful impulse undoubtedly colors my reflections here about my elder brother. Would Kevin have had an easier path, been less swept up in the tormenting tides of his adolescence – the head-strong rebelliousness, the addictions – if he and my parents had belonged to a more embracing and diverse extended family, one that might have better 'held' (Winnicott, 1960b) his unique stirrings at that time? The historical record here is far more ambiguous. Both my mother's elder brother and sister had sons who rejected college in favor of the trades, two as contractors, the third as a ship-builder (the latter, despite great success in his craft, struggled with alcoholism and died prematurely under circumstances reminiscent of Kevin's). In a development that would be unthinkable on the 'Indian' side of my extended family, however, where even second cousins are woven into the pattern of family life, these first cousins (and their parents) led lives that were completely removed from ours (I met two of the young men once in my childhood, but never laid eyes on the third). This culturally enforced, prototypically American sanding away of familial encumbrances – separation-individuation writ large, and the concomitant restricting of family to a kind of super-saturated, vertical relationship between parents and their progeny – deprived these young men and their parents of the kind of wide-ranging relational intercourse[8] that might have normalized their different pathways, and enabled their parents to see their underlying fealty to familial and cultural patterns buried beneath their rejection of the trappings of parental desires.

Within the literature of psychoanalysis and the mental health professions at large, of course, it has long been known that non-familial relationships – whether with teachers, therapists, neighbors or coaches, to say nothing of extended family members like aunts or grandparents, if sufficiently intimate (close by, familiar-quotidian) – can prove decisive in reversing the toxic effects of past trauma, while nurturing untapped areas of health and allowing teenagers to surmount seemingly insuperable obstacles. Unlike our still-dominant, ever more biologized discourse on adolescent development, however, this literature on resilience, like so much of contemporary writing on the analytic process, remains unfailingly 'relational' in focus, by which I mean that it sees selfhood as contextual, a biological fact whose shape and meaning are negotiated in the intimate, and widely variant overlap of expectations that frames families and cultures. This relational focus, applied to adolescence, can never free parents from the kind of worries that often characterize this phase of life, but does suggest a path toward understanding what the intimate 'point' of such struggles might be. Rather than only looking at remote factors – at the imponderables of hormones or genes, or the demands of the peer group or the dizzying impress of digital culture – parents, no less than psychotherapists, might benefit from trying to understand their teenagers in the context of what they see each morning when they look in the mirror: themselves, and the contradictory, at times impossible to fulfill welter of wishes and desires, both centrifugal and centripetal, that they bring to their children's process of growing up. In recognizing and perhaps getting help with these challenges – which of course aren't merely their own, but our culture's – parents may come to see that their teenagers' biggest and most intimate struggle in the adolescent passage is less about freeing themselves from parental expectations, but in finding a way (difficult as that can often seem) to fulfill them.

Notes

1 Not just for clinicians: Siegel's book, which includes an array of exercises targeting teenagers, will likely claim a corner on my 10-year-old's shelf in a few years' time.

2 Madame Metzinger was far from alone; Rimbaud's musical recapitulation of his opening in this stanza has had the same effect on me and countless others over the decades.

3 Glaring omissions – yet oddly consistent in the literature. Even Harold Benicsen's thoughtful, recent attachment-oriented interpretation (Bendicsen, 2013) – its cover emblazoned with the portrait of a solitary white male youth – takes that subset of teenagers as its baseline.

4 Clinicians schooled in the once-dominant ego psychological model of development (which Anna Freud shaped and to which Eric Erickson also contributed) will recall that Blos famously viewed the teenage years as a recapitulation of the stormy motoric and intrapsychic unfolding that occurs in first instance in toddlerhood. Margaret Mahler, the creator of the model of infant separation-individuation that inspired Blos (she coined the term), very much sought to describe a universal epigenesis, one that stands outside of culture. In the pages that follow, I walk in the footsteps of many others who have sought to draw attention to the very specific, far from universal assumptions and biases woven into this theory (see, for example, Galatzer-Levy & Cohler, 1990, 1993; Akhtar & Kramer, 1998).

5 I use the words "American" and "Indian" here as a convenient shorthand to denote the cultural origin of the different sides of the family, though my husband's side (aka, the "Indian side") includes both American citizens (first or second generation) and citizens of India.

6 I am aware that this picture of South Asian adolescence is a rosy one and that it neglects some of the downsides of an omnipresent, ritually involved extended family. The relational demands of the broader system can be a special trial, for example, for daughters-in-law contending with their husbands' (co-habituating, at times dictatorial) parents, and are manifest as well in the subtler but no less striking lack of "personal space" on the subcontinent (and that many South Asians like my in-laws view as a welcome facet of the North American experience). Notwithstanding these limitations, the culture of family life within the South Asian context also has many strengths, some of which are highlighted in this discussion, and which have often been under-emphasized or pathologized in psychoanalytic accounts.

7 Or even as a word: Baxter (2008) notes that the term 'adolescence' only entered the English language in the mid-19th century, with 'teenager' coming even later – in the 1930s.

8 Not just vertical connections between parents and children, but lateral (siblings, cousins) and diagonal (grandparents, aunts/uncles, nieces and nephews, etc.).

Chapter 4

Friendship, friendliness and intimacy

Gurmeet Kanwal

Let's start with the observation that the first letter of the word 'intimacy' is 'I'. Curiously, if we look at the first two letters, we get the word 'in', and the first three letters provide us with a clue to the Latin derivation of the word from the root word 'intimus' (Wiktionary, 2018), implying 'innermost'. How is it then that we have come to regard intimacy in psychology as a subject having to do with closeness *between* people?

Here is one way to understand this. The extent to which one has the possibility of establishing intimacy with another person depends on the extent to which one is connected to one's own innermost subjectivity in a full and wholesome manner. Intimacy becomes a phenomenon between people, but only by having its origin in the experience of intimacy with one's self. Too often, one sees in clinical work people who are desperately trying to establish relationships (intimacy) with others while not having established an intimacy with their own subjectivity. The more prevalent dissociative operations are in a self system, the harder it is to have a fully satisfying relational experience. While dissociations are sometimes the only way to survive relational trauma, "As a proactive way of living, however, the subsequent cost of this solution to each individual is always identical – to one degree or another, an unlived life" (Bromberg, 1998, p. 202) – and hence an unloved one too!

The opposite is also true. The way one gets to experience intimacy with one's own subjectivity is by encountering it in a relational setting. Developmentally this begins with the mother/caretaker-infant dyad and proceeds from there to larger and larger relational circles.

So this is how the intrapsychic and interpersonal are perpetually and developmentally linked – through recursive experiential dynamics where the relational constantly constructs the personal, and the personal constantly generates the relational. Disruptions in one lead to disruptions in the other. The intrapsychic and the interpersonal are completely dependent on each other, or to put it another way, they are completely interdependent. Or as Bromberg (1998) puts it, "a continuing negotiation between the two subjective realities of creative interiority and social relatedness" (p. 127).

Hence intimacy is a circular experience that can either be seen as beginning from one's innermost being and proceeding outward to establish relationships, or it can be seen as proceeding from a relational context that allows the development and experience of one's subjectivity. What theoretical model one uses depends on where one wants to put one's metapsychological finger in tracing the surface of this Mobius strip. There are not two surfaces being traced by the one finger here, other than by virtue of a perceptual illusion. It is all one interpersonal/intrapsychic surface. A couplet by a 15th-century Indian poet, Kabir, states it well, with the first line translated as, "The street of love is so narrow that two cannot pass through it".[1] The psychological implication of the couplet can be used as a metaphor for the etymology of 'intimacy'. Being in love implies there are two, and yet in a paradoxical way, there is only room for one. The interpersonal perspective implies two, the intrapsychic perspective implies one. But the paradox (not to be resolved, as Winnicott would warn us) is that they are both one and the same, originating within a seamless circularity. Thus the word 'intimacy' makes both etymological and psychological sense. One particular kind of experience of relatedness and intimacy, that is not talked about enough in psychoanalytic literature, is friendliness. This chapter is about the relationship between friendliness and intimacy. Where do we place friendliness in a psychanalytic context? What is its value, developmentally, psychodynamically and clinically, in understanding and facilitating intimacy?

In his introduction to *Playing and Reality* (1971), Winnicott wrote, "In considering the place of these phenomena in the life of a child one must recognize the central position of Winnie the Pooh;" It is curious that 27 years later Winnie the Pooh was anointed and honored as the global mascot of friendship by the United Nations. What did Winnicott's reference to Winnie the Pooh imply? Perhaps Winnicott was intuitively pointing to the significance of friendships as much as he was to the significance of transitional objects and play, although he said little about friendship in particular. In 1998, the UN General Assembly honored Pooh Bear and family with a commemorative inscription thanking him for his consistent message of "companionship, loyalty and friendship to the world". United Nations also proclaimed July 30 as the 'International Day of Friendship' in 2011. Whether it be through books, poetry, folklore or film, the world has always recognized the importance of friendship in human life, far more than we psychoanalysts ever have, at least in our theories.

Definitions

Aristotle has been quoted by many writers considering the topic of friendship. This is because in his seminal work, *Nicomachean Ethics*, he elaborates three kinds of friendships. Thompson (1998) summarizes Aristotle's categories as, "(1) friends who offer a source of pleasure; (2) friends with whom we engage in commerce; and finally (3) those friends whom we love simply for being themselves" (pp. 553–554). However, this chapter is not about types of friendship, but rather an attempt to get behind the psychoanalytic understanding of friendliness as a psychic experience and affect. To keep that clarity, I would suggest the following definitions:

Friendship is a relational equation dominated by an attitude of friendliness that becomes consolidated over time so that the advantages of maintaining the relational equation begin to outweigh many other social demands, desires or obligations. Often, particularly at certain developmental stages, this can even take precedence over sexual desires – "Bros before Hos" or "Chicks before Dicks" are rallying cries for such homosocial (in this case non-sexual) priorities. Kayleen Schaefer (2018) explores this centrality of woman to woman friendship in her book, *Text Me When You Get Home: The Evolution and Triumph of Modern Female Friendship*. Similarly, Michael Kimmel elaborates this dynamic for guys in his book, *Guyland* (2008), stating, "Masculinity is largely a 'homosocial' experience: performed for, and judged by, other men" (p. 47).

Friends are individuals able to sustain friendship over significant periods of time. Friends are not acquaintances or colleagues or family, although friendliness can be found in all of those relationships, and often there may be overlap between those categories. One cultural and philologically noxious effect of Facebook, in my opinion, has been the perversion of the word 'friend', by implying that anyone who happens to make it to your Facebook page is designated a 'friend'. The word 'friend' has taken on a meaning in the digital world that is illusory, ephemeral and misleading. Additionally, it takes the centrally cooperative principle underlying friendliness and converts it into a competitive and commercial one, with people vying to have a bigger 'number' than the next person on their 'friend' list.

While friendship is the ongoing relational state between two friends, **friendliness** is a state of relational integration between people that has to be seen as *dynamic*. That is, it is constantly changing, appearing and disappearing, forming and dissolving, becoming dormant or active, in any relational setting, whether it be between 'friends' or lovers, or spouses, or even parents and children, and also between patients and therapists (transferentially or otherwise).

There is a distinction between intimacy and friendliness that is important to keep in mind. Intimacy is value neutral. It can be 'good' or 'bad'. Intimacy can become structured around malevolence, hostility or aggression – i.e. some people can be involved in a sadomasochistic intimacy. That sort of intimacy involves a continuous fluctuation between conjunctive and disjunctive (Sullivanian terms that I will return to later) motivations – like schizoid phenomena where the fluctuation is between avoidance and approach. We can see intimacy between partners where one is abusive and the other abused, or where one is exploitative and the other exploited, or where one is the oppressor and the other oppressed, or where one is committed and loyal while the other is unfaithful and deceptive. In many of these circumstances we can find ourselves wondering, why are they still together? Often our patients are in treatment exactly to figure that out for themselves.

Friendliness, on the other hand, in my view, always refers to a positive element of intimacy. Friendliness is never 'bad' or pathological or maladaptive. We can have bad friends, just like we can have bad partners or spouses or lovers. But I am suggesting that friendliness is that aspect of relating that refers to concern for the other (Winnicott, 1963), interpersonal security (Sullivan, 1953), playfulness rather than libidinal fulfillment (Winnicott, 1971), and cooperation rather than competitiveness (Majolo, Ames, & Brumpton, 2006). Friends can be competitive, but friendliness is that quality between them that is non-competitive. This distinction has not usually been made in the psychological literature on friendship and friendliness. Friendliness is not libidinal attachment minus something, it is not 'aim-inhibited' drive (Freud, 1921), rather, it is an aim in its own right. Friendliness is not a way station on an interrupted journey to sexual fulfillment, or a detouring sublimation of aggressive, competitive wishes and fantasies. Friendliness is a product of behavioral and psychological evolution that ensures survival through cooperation, affiliation, relaxation and security. That is why we see it in humans as well as animals. The absence of this clarity is largely responsible for the dearth of psychoanalytic literature on friendliness, starting with Freud's subsumption of it under Drive Theory.

Friendliness and Drive Theory

Between the libidinal/sexual drive fueling intimacy, and the aggressive/thanatophillic drive disrupting or perverting it, where, if anywhere, did Freud visualize a space for the psychological need and characteristics for friendship? Not really anywhere. In Freud's words, "friendship or friendliness is aim-inhibited sexuality or aim-inhibited love" (Freud, 1921). In his binary perspective, all seemingly non-drive driven interactions were reducible to one or the other. All human activities were, for Freud, masked, drive derivatives and compromise formations. If one accepts that premise, then there is not much to be said about friendship beyond uncovering its rootedness in a sublimated form of drive satisfaction where both aggression and libido are constrained in certain ways, creating some room for an interaction that tends to be (therefore) relatively conflict-free. However this view of friendship and friendliness purloins the possibility of understanding a human experience that is ubiquitous, essential and yet mostly neglected in psychoanalytic thinking.

Leo Rangell (1963), describing Freud's opinion of friendship, quotes a personal communication with Hart, referring to his (Hart's) statement that "friendliness and friendship are referred to as if they were dilute editions of love, much as pink is regarded as a dilution of red". Radomisli (1968), focusing on the aim-inhibition of aggression rather than libido, writes, "It is perhaps time, then, to re-examine the psychoanalytic theory of friendship and to question whether aim-inhibited aggression is not as important in friendship as aim-inhibited sexuality". Both Rangell and Radomisli thus continue the Freudian formulation of friendship and friendliness as 'aim-inhibited' expressions of libidinal or aggressive drives. In this chapter I present a viewpoint that is quite the opposite of that. I will point to some alternative possibilities, primarily anchored in an interpersonal/relational theoretical tradition. I will argue that friendliness deserves its own chromatic home in the spectral neighborhood of relational possibilities.

What is the evidence against friendship being a sublimated form of libidinal activity? All kinds of people have friends – those who are libidinally quite free and satisfied, as well as those who are libidinally conflicted and repressed. But their friendships don't necessarily show consistently different characteristics. There are some people who have a lot of trouble making friends. These people often also have trouble with romantic/sexual relationships. And for the people who have trouble with sexuality, but not much problem with friendship, their capacity for friendship does not seem to change as their sexual issues get resolved. They still have the same need to have friends. In many societies, lack of filial connections (leading to social alienation or humiliation) can be much more devastating than the lack of capacity to have sexual intimacy. In other words cultures may value friendliness above sexual intimacy.

We also know from time immemorial that friendships can cross all sorts of established human social barriers. Cross socioeconomic and cross caste friendships have been described even in ancient Indian myths, e.g. Krishna (of royal lineage and a manifestation of divinity) and Sudama (a poor and humble villager); and Karna (mistakenly presumed at the time to be of lower caste) and Duryodhana (a prince, hence of upper caste) in the Mahabharata. In Melville's Moby Dick we witness the unlikely friendship between Ishmael and Queequeg, one being pulled to the other against all odds, "Wild he was; a very sight of sights to see; yet I began to see myself mysteriously drawn toward him" (p. 44). Friendships between potential sexual partners seem to be a bigger challenge in popular literature. The classic example is seen in the movie *When Harry met Sally* (released in 1989). Despite their best efforts, and much arguing about the possibility of friendship, the two protagonists end up as lovers. The conclusion is that friendliness between potential sexual partners easily leads to sexual intimacy. But if friendly intimacy can become the road to sexual intimacy, then how can friendliness be 'aim-inhibited' sexuality? Is it a road or a road block? Friendliness facilitates sexuality; it is not a detour from sexuality. Certainly not in any universal sense.

We see cross-species friendliness (a dog is considered man's best friend) even when we do not see cross-species sexual reproduction. In fact the defining feature of a species is the lack of cross-species reproductive possibility. However, there is abundant evidence of cross-species friendliness. Interestingly images of cross-species friendliness hold a tremendous appeal for humans. Jennifer Holland's book, *Unlikely Friendships* (Holland, 2011), with 47 stories of cross-species friendliness is popular enough to rank #304 on Amazon's Kindle list. There may be many reasons for this reaction. I will suggest three here, while it is certainly possible that there may be others: (i) These images demonstrate that one need not be afraid of things (or feelings, e.g. of aggression) that one has habitually been afraid of – like an image of friendship between a tiger and a goat, or watching a bird peck food out of a crocodile's teeth! (ii) Witnessing cross-species friendliness falls within the realm of breaking taboos, and as such, it holds an ontogenic fascination for us. These taboos may not only be about sexuality or incestuality. They may also be taboos that underlie xenophobia and many of our prejudices.

(iii) There is an inherent optimism in the possibility of cross-species friendliness. Implied is the notion that drives can be tamed, deep seated evolutionary obstacles overcome, dissociated elements of one's mind co-exist, and even become integrated. Cross-species friendliness thus kindles the power of the Ideal. This biological and evolutionary phenomenon of cross-species friendliness has just not been taken into account in psychoanalytic thinking on friendliness or friendship. Cross-species friendship is also what makes Winnie the Pooh and his group of friends (a bear, a pig, two kangaroos, a donkey, a tiger, a rabbit, an owl, and even a human) so delightful to children and adults alike.

While it is true that libidinal and aggressive impulses might be *practiced within*, or *displaced into*, an interpersonal field integrated around friendliness, this does not mean that friendliness is present simply to allow such expression. It does not logically imply that friendliness is 'aim-inhibited' instinctual activity. It simply means that because interpersonal security is a relational characteristic of friendliness, and because play is ontogenetically associated with it, friendships can often safely survive the expression of aggressive and even eroticized elements. How much libidinal and aggressive expression friendships can safely contain varies from culture to culture, and dyad to dyad. And within any given culture what is allowed between men is different than what is allowed between women (Rubin, 1986). When I compare my experience of growing up in India with living in the U.S., for example, I am struck by the much greater latitude friendships between men are allowed in terms of emotional warmth, touching and verbal affection. Similar behavior in the U.S. is much more likely to be seen as evidence of homosexual leanings. However, it is precisely that kind of culture-bound interpretation that can make friendliness seem like "aim-inhibited sexuality". Schaffner (2001) describing his experience of being in India makes the same observation, "Westerners traveling in India are often surprised to see men walking along the streets, arm in arm or linking fingers as a sign of friendship, not as a sign of homosexual interest" (p. 119).

While being groundbreaking in addressing the topic, Rangell's (1963) paper on friendliness has two problems: it fails to maintain the distinction between investigating friendliness as an *affective/relational state* and friendship as a *relational structure*, and, while recognizing the early origin of friendliness, its roots in play and transitional object experience and its relationship to security (as counterpoint to anxiety), it fails to see the flaw in Freud's logic regarding 'aim-inhibition' of drives as the primary function of friendship.

Evidence of friendliness as a *primary* developmental path and capacity can also be seen in the significance of play. We know from a variety of fields of study – psychoanalysis, cognitive science, sociology, anthropology, biology – that play is central to the wellbeing of socially oriented organisms, as well as universal across species and cultures (Bekoff, 1998; Bekoff & Jessica, 2009; Brown & Christopher, 2009; Burghardt, 2005; Smith, 1982). We know that play starts early and continues throughout life. However, because we can see elements of aggressive and libidinal expression in various forms of play does not logically imply that play is simply 'aim-inhibited' sexuality or aggression. Neither does it imply that the evolution of play has occurred in order to divert or manage libidinal and aggressive drive impulses. Correlation is not causality.

In fact I would suggest that it is often the other way around. Eroticism can often become a misdirected attempt to satisfy one's need for friendship and friendliness. This creates problems in the romantic area of the relationship. The task of therapy then is to free the desire for friendship of its contamination with eroticism. I find patients who have suffered sexual abuse in childhood to often have trouble discriminating between the two. Friendliness in their developmental experience may become corrupted and perverted by the abusive parent's uncontrolled eroticism. One such young woman who identified as bisexual had trouble keeping friends because sooner or later she would either end up sleeping with them, or she would become angry at what she perceived to be erotic desires of the other person intruding into her wish to keep it at the level of a friendship. She then perceived her 'friends' to be exploitative and selfish. What we understood was that friendliness made her anxious and insecure because she could not be sure that it would stick. She 'needed' sexual contact (she thought) to become certain of the other person's interest in her. And yet as soon as sexuality intervened it became much harder to know what the interest was really about. The fantasied solution became another problem, and the real solution kept eluding her.

In fact there are multiple theories to account for why play has evolved in animals, and there is no overarching agreement in the general scientific literature. Pellis, Pellis and Bell (2010) classify existing theories into two main categories: "the motor training hypothesis" and "training for the unexpected" hypothesis. The motor training hypothesis implies that play is a way to train the organism's body as well as brain to engage in adult behaviors. The authors point to evidence in changes noted in the areas of the cerebellum that control motor behavior, for instance. In fact it appears that, "different types of play peak at different times during the infancy of monkeys and that these peaks correspond to the times at which different – and presumably associated – brain areas mature" (p. 281). The second hypothesis implies that the unpredictability and variability in play behavior is a way for the organism to develop greater competency in dealing with the unpredictable and the unexpected in life. Accordingly, "Play is a means of exposing an animal to new situations and of its testing new behaviors" (p. 282). They then go on to suggest a third possibility that might be able to subsume the two others: "Play trains animals to be resilient by modifying the neural circuitry that regulates emotional responses" (p. 292). The scientific data point to play as a multifunctional activity that is neither a diversion of sexual impulses, nor limited to practicing components of adult sexual behavior.

Among psychoanalysts, Winnicott was the one to create a new kind of space within which to conceptualize developmental aspects of play. By positing the concept of potential space and transitional phenomena, Winnicott delinked play from drives, and elaborated a developmental line from infancy into adulthood for various activities in the creative sphere, all of which he referred to as 'play', including the experience of psychoanalytic treatment. He states very explicitly, "But playing needs to be studied on its own, supplementary to the concept of the sublimation of instinct. It may very well be that we have missed something by having these two phenomena (playing and masturbatory activity) so closely linked in our minds. I have tried to point out that when a child is playing the masturbatory element is essentially lacking" (p. 39). Further along he writes, "It must be of value to the analyst to be constantly reminded not only of what is owed to Freud but also of what we owe to the natural and universal thing called playing" (p. 41). I find this to be a startling statement whose implications classical theory has yet to fully digest or admit. Following Winnicott's observation, I am suggesting that play is not possible without the affect of friendliness, and that therefore, friendliness, like play, needs to be understood separate from aim-inhibition of drives. Winnicott ends his paper with the following statement, "Playing is inherently exciting and precarious. This characteristic derives not from instinctual arousal but from the precariousness that belongs to the interplay in the child's mind of that which is subjective (near hallucination) and that which is objectively perceived (actual, or shared reality)" (p. 52).

Rangell admits to the significance of Winnicott's ideas of transitional phenomena (which for Winnicott leads into the space of play) in understanding friendliness. He writes, "I might mention as an early 'friend' the transitional object described by Winnicott. There may be a blanket, or a pet, or a rag doll". He goes on to say, "It then comes to serve as an early, if not a first, 'friend', an external adjunct to a tender and inexperienced ego in its struggle to master the helpless state" (p. 15). He also writes (sounding like Sullivan), "The same considerations apply and the same prerequisites exist for the development of anxiety, of which, by the way, the affect of friendliness is a counterpart" (p. 13). However, despite his insight into the connection between friendliness and security (counterpoint to anxiety), and between friendliness and transitional phenomena (and therefore, by implication, play), he finds it hard to go against the established classical notion of friendliness as arising out of aim-inhibition of drives. Winnicott, on the other hand, saw it as a form of 'ego-relatedness', stating, "It will be seen that I attach great importance to this relationship, as I consider that it is the stuff out of which friendship is made" (Winnicott, 1958, p. 33).

Interpersonal developmental understanding of friendliness

For Sullivan the shape of any interpersonal interaction is all about establishing a sense of security. The various mechanisms people use to bring this about are therefore termed 'security operations' (Sullivan, 1953). Developmentally this need for security begins at birth with the attention to physical 'needs' like hunger. The behavior and feeling triggered in the caretaking person by the infant's needs is referred to as 'tenderness'. Tenderness was defined by Sullivan as, "a certain tension, . . . which is a potentiality for or an illusion to activities suited to – or more or less suited to – the general relief of the infant's needs" (p. 40). Thus the tension of hunger is relieved (Sullivan calls this 'satisfaction') by the tenderness of the mother providing her breast. Sullivan then hypothesizes that unlike the tension of physical needs which is related to the infant's "physico-chemical environment", the tension of *anxiety* is entirely a function of "communal existence with a personal environment. The relaxation of the tension of anxiety . . . is the experience not of satisfaction, but of interpersonal *security*" (p. 42). Security and self-worth, or self-esteem, are the key components of mental health for Sullivan. The capacity for intimacy rests on these attributes. Sullivan (1953) writes, "Intimacy is that type of situation involving two people which permits validation of all components of self-worth" (pp. 245–248).

The notions of 'relaxation' and 'interpersonal security' are also closely related to the development and dynamics of friendliness. These same relational characteristic are essential to the activity of play. Play gets disrupted if libidinal demands or expectations intrude in a non-mutual fashion. The same is true for friendliness. According to interpersonal theory then, friendliness can be seen as a developmental acquisition of an adequate amount of security, self-worth and satisfaction. The foundations of this capacity begin to be laid during infancy, and then there are certain developmental stages where the exercise of this capacity becomes central and can lead to the establishment of long-term friendships, or as Sullivan referred to it – 'chumship'. As Weinberg (1989) put it, "It is an interpersonal process that provides the kind of consensual validation that is so necessary a part of intimacy, that Sullivan underscored it in his discussion of the preadolescent era as a key factor in the development of interpersonal integration and a true sense of self, through chumship". For Sullivan the establishment of 'chumship' had the potential of protecting against significant disturbances, such as a schizophrenic process.

In order to understand friendliness in the context of interpersonal meta psychology, it is also necessary to take into account Sullivan's (1953) notions of 'conjunctive' and 'disjunctive' dynamisms (a 'dynamism' being a pattern of interaction). 'Conjunctive' dynamisms are those that are relatively free of anxiety, and work to enhance security as well as intimacy. 'Disjunctive' dynamisms are ones that are shaped by significant interpersonal anxiety, making it hard for the individuals to feel secure, and they lead one away from the possibility of intimacy. A particularly noxious form of a disjunctive dynamism is what Sullivan referred to as 'malevolent transformation'. This is a situation where an individual is so anxious about the interaction that he or she both expects malevolence and, in anticipation, reacts with malevolence, thus subverting any possibility of intimacy. Friendliness, as I understand it, is always a conjunctive dynamism. It is very much the opposite of malevolent transformation. Elsewhere, in a different context, I have referred to this possibility of a dynamism that actively increases the chance of the interaction remaining conjunctive as a 'benevolent transformation' (Kanwal, 2017) as opposed to a malevolent transformation. While friendliness was not my focus there, I would now consider friendliness as another form of benevolent transformation.

The experience of adequate tenderness during infancy lays the groundwork for the possibility of an adequate sense of security and hence increases the likelihood of satisfactory conjunctive interactions as life moves on. These conjunctive tendencies are a necessary condition for the successful development of one's capacity for friendliness, as well as for one's capacity for sexual and romantic relationships. However the point I am emphasizing is that friendliness is a separate (and equally important) developmental path from the sexual/romantic, and not, as Freud (and Klein) suggested, either a sublimation or inhibition of libidinal impulses. Relational psychoanalytic theory gives us a better way of understanding friendliness than classical theory did. Relational theory allows us to formulate that friendliness is a state of mind which facilitates the integration of dissociated self-states (Bromberg writes, in Chefetz & Bromberg, 2004, "Get to know your Not-Me's. Some of my own Not-Me's have become very close friends, over time"), because it is a relational equation of security and relaxation. The understanding of the centrality of security and friendliness is important on a macro sociocultural level as well.

Friendliness and xenophobia

All over the world today we see the manifestations and consequences of xenophobia. Psychologically speaking, if xenophobia is to be understood as the anxiety or fear one experiences in the presence of that which is unfamiliar, foreign, dissimilar, from elsewhere or simply 'other', then the attitude and affect of friendliness is its exact psychological antonym. In that sense, in a geopolitical atmosphere where "xenophobic nationalism" (Akhtar, 2017), parochialism and jingoism are becoming pervasive, it has become increasingly important to understand the corresponding diminishment of friendliness. If friendliness is emergent from a sense of security and conjunctive relational capacities, the current atmosphere of insecurity and terror makes disjunctive tendencies dominant, thus making it difficult for friendliness to thrive. This then begins the vicious cycle of increasing alienation between fellow human beings. Akhtar (2007) refers to the incapacity to even think about the ways one person alienates the other as "unmentalized xenophobia". If we understand the deep and foundational significance of friendliness in psychological development, and in our ability to play, we can see how fundamentally devastating and potentially dangerous the current trends are. Not just for our political and economic health, but for the psychological health of the generations growing up in these times. "Unmentalized xenophobia" makes friendliness impossible. In an iconic scene in the movie *Forrest Gump* (released in 1994), Forrest as a disabled young boy getting on the school bus for the first time resolves the dilemma of strangeness by the simple act of introducing himself to the driver and having her introduce herself to him. "Now we ain't strangers anymore", he says. It is remarkable how often we all fail to take that simple step towards friendliness in our personal, professional as well as political lives.

Ciaramelli (2001), in his elegant essay on friendship and desire, elaborates La Boetie's thesis about the nature of friendship being antithetical to the desire for domination. In Ciaramelli's view, "La Boétie initially concludes that the principle of domination renders friendship impossible" (p. 373). Friendliness is the foundation for democracy. Derrida (1993) makes this clear to us while investigating the mourning underlying his opening statement in "Politics of friendship", "O my friends, there is no friend" – a phrase attributed to Aristotle by Montaigne. Derrida writes,

> If the great canonical meditations on friendship (Cicero's De amicitia, Montaigne's De l'amitié, Blanchot's L'amitié, for example) belong to the experience of mourning, to the moment of loss – that of the friend or of friendship – if, through the irreplaceable element of the name, they always advance into the testamentary shadow in order to *entrust and refuse* the death of the unique one to a universalizable discourse. . .
>
> (p. 385)

then perhaps it is this friendship that is the basis of justice, and it is in its absence that we feel the absence of democracy. Derrida ends by asking, "When will we be ready for an experience of equality that would be a respectful test of this friendship, and that would at last be just, just beyond justice as law, that is, measure up to its immea-sure?" (p. 388).

I would suggest, extending Derrida, that as the space for *play* (and hence friendliness) diminishes in a society, so does the possibility of justice, equality and democracy. When competition, domination, greed, envy and xenophobia begin to overshadow friendliness and cooperation we have the beginnings of the end of a civilization. The dissociative gaps within individuals and between people begin to increase, systems become more rigid, thinking becomes concrete, and what is 'not-me' is seen as worthy of extermination. This convergent consequence of dissociative anxieties within oneself, and the dissociative anxieties between members of a community or between different ethnic, racial, cultural, national groups has been well explicated by Kristeva (1994) in her book *Strangers to Oneself*. Bromberg (2011) (as well as Allan Schore in his foreword to Bromberg's book) makes the point that this psychological disaster can also be documented in our biology, "The more intense the unsymbolized affect, the more powerful the dissociative forces that prevent isolated islands of selfhood from becoming linked within working memory" (p. 79).

A large amount of psychoanalytic literature is accumulating on the topic of 'otherness' in clinical work as well as theoretical frameworks. This has natural implications for intimacy in various forms. One area that has not received enough attention in relation to otherness is the notion of friendliness as *the developmental foundation that determines how any individual handles otherness*, whether it be in the form of racism, sexism, nationalism or any other destructive -ism. I believe when early relational trauma leads to difficulties in acquiring the capacity for friendliness (an extreme case being what Sullivan describes as "malevolent transformation") it sets the stage for difficulties in dealing with 'otherness'. Friendliness is antithetical to stranger-ness. The capacity for friendliness is an essential developmental acquisition for the possibility of avoiding an extreme and rigid boundedness that makes mistrust, prejudice and xenophobia more likely to flourish in a personality and a community. In that sense it evokes the Eriksonian stage of "Trust vs. Mistrust", as well as Balint's idea of "Basic Fault" vs. "basic trust". Friendliness is based on trust, just as play is. Mistrust, on the other hand is associated with "Basic Fault" (Balint, 1968), or that which is not-known, foreign, dissociated or 'not-me'. Pervasive dissociation of 'not-me' leads to the dangerous ubiquity of 'not-you'.

Clinical notes/friendship as transference

Once we can correct the notion that friendliness is "aim-inhibited sexuality" it becomes possible to look at the unique characteristics of friendliness as it might appear in a therapeutic situation – both in the transference-countertransference framework, as well as when it manifests as a function of the 'real' relationship between patient and therapist. Patients do bring in their experiences of friendship all the time in therapy. However, I think therapists could do more in having friendliness on their minds as a capacity worth assessing, noticing, working with and inquiring about. It would be good for candidates and psychiatric residents and other kinds of clinical students to be taught to pay attention to this dynamic. The capacity for friendliness is a good prognostic indicator for establishing a productive therapeutic alliance. In Winnicott's (1958) words, "It may turn out to be the matrix of transference" (p. 33).

One of the most noxious effects of traumatic experience in early childhood is that it sets the child apart from peers. It creates a sense of belonging to a different world. The shame accompanying relational trauma often makes it impossible for these kids to establish friendships, or have adequate opportunities to express their capacities for friendliness. The aloneness that results is often even more dangerous than the pain of the trauma, which realization I owe particularly to one of my very traumatized patients. Had it not been for a couple of friends he was able to find in childhood he might very well have not survived abuse at the hands of a psychotic mother and a manifestly evil father. In our work together also, elements of friendship and friendliness became a very important part of the relationship. The usual stance when patients express a desire to be 'friends' with their therapist is to interpret the desire as either a resistance to becoming aware of eroticized elements or to the continuation of the treatment, or an acting out meant to break the frame, or a reaction formation against repressed hostility. Weinberg (1989) writes,

> We always take note when they view us as possible lovers. But do we miss the moment when they see us as chums? Does it register and if so how do we respond when they see us as friends? What does it mean in the therapy when

> their view of us shifts from Mahler's "reference point" to Bowlby's "one who stands behind"? It may be that it is more threatening to us to be viewed as a "trusted companion" than as the protective or authoritarian parentified figure, or longed for lover we so quickly interpret. Yet in many ways when our patients begin to see us in this way, could it not be the clearest signal of all that the distance between the analyst and the patient has actually lessened? And it is this, the closeness, the directness, the egalitarianism which threatens us more than it does the patient as it presents us with that "who me?" feeling. Oddly, this happens when we have achieved something of what we have worked for in the analysis.
>
> (p. 364)

Guy-Thompson (1998), while staying true to the idea of friendship as "aim-inhibited" love, makes a case for the analytic relationship having the same characteristics as friendship. He goes on to state, "In effect, the transference neurosis is a form of friendship, manifested by the trials of aim-inhibited love" (p. 559). Freud (1937, p. 222) on the other hand, writes, "not every good relationship between an analyst and his subject during and after analysis was to be regarded as a transference; there were also friendly relations which were based on reality and which proved to be viable". I like the way Weinberg (1989) puts it, "The analyst can be, and is, an 'ambassador' of friendship for the patient".

Another traumatized patient came in years ago specifically to deal with the grief of losing a pet. She much preferred having animals as friends to people. Animals were safer, they were not likely to disappoint, they did not need to misunderstand. It was very important for her to have created this space for the experience of friendliness, even if within the animal world.

In one of my supervisions, when I was in training, I had the good fortune of having a supervisor point out to me that I was jumping to interpret a particular moment of a patient's transference as being an expression of latent homosexuality, when in fact to my supervisor it seemed to be all about wanting me as a friend. This made historical sense for this patient who had suffered the loss of a friend early in life.

Another category of patients to consider is immigrants who often come in mourning the loss of opportunities to exercise their capacity for friendliness, and the absence of longstanding friendships left behind in some far away place. In my experience this is a very common reason for depression in immigrants. Not the difficulty in finding the intimacy of romance as much as the difficulty in finding the intimacy of friendship. I think it is to this need that we owe the vast proliferation of platforms and apps that provide a sense of connectedness and friendships. For those who are separated at a particular time in their life from friends they grew up with, the task of making new friends in a new cultural environment can be quite daunting (Ainslie et al., 2013). Sometimes the analyst may function as a friendship-bridge between the immigrant and the host culture, enabling the patient to become more secure in the possibility of exercising friendliness. If the therapist does not recognize the uniqueness of friendliness as a developmental path and a psychic need, he or she may interpret along the lines of 'aim-inhibited' sexuality, thus missing an important therapeutic need and opportunity.

Conclusion

Making the mistake of understanding friendliness as simply an 'aim-inhibited' state diminishes its contribution to psychological health and development, as well as its role in social and global affairs. In this chapter I have tried to emphasize the uniqueness, as well as the foundational developmental significance, of friendliness as a psychic experience. Friendliness is associated with interpersonal security, relaxation and play. It is from that perspective, not one of sexuality, that the clinical significance of friendliness must be understood, approached and interpreted. Understanding friendliness in this way might also have the effect of freeing psychoanalysts to see, facilitate and accept the presence of friendliness in the transference-countertransference/enactment matrix. When we look around at this time we see a sea change in the ways that intimacy is being explored by people around the world. Whether it be heterosexual or homosexual intimacy, or polyamory, or intimacy across the borders of race, ethnicity and culture, or across age differences and gender spectrums, the psychoanalytic emphasis tends to be on what is happening sexually. What is not attended to is what all of this can help us understand about the centrality of friendliness and friendships. One frequently hears people talk about having or wanting 'friends with benefits' (of being lovers). There may be times, however, when what they really need is 'lovers with benefits' (of being friends).

Note

1 In Hindi: "Prem gali ati sankri tame do na samaye".

Chapter 5

Intimacy and otherness in multicultural/interracial/interfaith couples

Bari Smelson-Kanwal

Introduction

As a psychoanalyst and couples therapist working in New York City and Westchester County, my practice is filled with a diverse group of people. As a white Jewish female who is in a multicultural, interracial, interfaith heterosexual relationship, a substantial percentage of my colleagues send me couples and individuals who are multicultural, interracial and/or interfaith. Having spent more than 25 years living, pondering and working with the issues that affect couples that don't share similar ethnicity, race, culture, class or religion I have been drawn to understand what works and doesn't work in these relationships. In this chapter, I will discuss the issues pertaining to couples that have these differences and describe some common factors that I observe in their pursuit of psychic intimacy. I will also outline three cases representing composites that illustrate the difficulties that can crop up and suggest how a couples therapist can enhance intimacy when couple conflicts stem from feelings of otherness, loss, loneliness, guilt and societal oppression. In my experience these issues are important to look for in the psychic lives of multicultural, interracial and interfaith couples.

The term multicultural refers to individuals having several cultural or ethnic backgrounds. Interracial couples are those where the individuals represent one or more racial groups. Interfaith couples encompass two or more religions. The literature defines these kinds of relationships as intercultural, interracial, multicultural, cross-cultural or multiethnic. Race and ethnicity have been used to mean the same thing. Killian (2017) states,

> Ethnicity may be differentiated from race in that it refers to a sense of common heritage made up of similarities of religion, history and national or geographic origin. Ethnicity is linked to one's social and familial legacies and traditions. . ., race is closely linked to biology and physiognomy.
>
> (p. 232)

Multicultural couples may also be interracial and or interfaith. In this paper, I will refer to such couples by using the acronym MII, implying multicultural, interracial or interfaith couples as a group.

Changing statistics

There has been a substantial increase in the number of multicultural and interracial couples cohabitating and marrying in the United States. A Pew Research Center study (2017) found that in 2015, 17% of all U.S. marriages were interracial, "a more than fivefold increase from 3% in 1967". According to Wang (Pew Research Center, 2015), "Of the 3.6 million adults who got married in 2013, 58% of American Indians, 28% of Asians, 19% of blacks and 7% of whites have a spouse whose race was different from their own". The Pew Research Center (2017) also reported that in 2015,

> Nearly three-in-ten Asian newlyweds (29%) were married to someone of a different race or ethnicity . . . as were 27% of Hispanic newlyweds. Intermarriage for these groups was especially prevalent among the U.S. born: 39% of U.S.-born Hispanics and almost half (46%) of U.S.-born Asian newlyweds were intermarried in 2015.

Further,

> Four-in-ten newlyweds in Honolulu (42%) are married to someone of a different race or ethnicity, followed by newlyweds living in the Las Vegas (31%) and Santa Barbara, California (30%) metro areas. At the same time, just 3% of newlyweds in or around Asheville, North Carolina, and Jackson, Mississippi, are intermarried.
>
> (Pew Research Center, 2017)

More specifically, in 2015, 42% of Hispanics, 15% of Asians and 11% of African Americans were married to a white spouse (Livingston & Brown, 2017). "In the same year, 24% of recently married black men were intermarried, compared with 12% of newly married black women" (Bialik, 2017). However, whites are marrying out of their race at a lower rate (Livingston & Brown, 2017). Overall, interracial marriages are seen as being less stable than endogamous marriages (Zhang & Van Hook, 2009). The more highly educated, however, the less likely they are to get a divorce.

A Pew Research Center analysis of the U.S. Census Bureau states that 18% of cohabitating adults have a partner of a different race or ethnicity. Millennials and Gen Xers are more likely to have this arrangement with 46% of Asian adults living with individuals from a different race or ethnicity. The statistic combines 38% of immigrants and 59% U.S.-born Asian individuals (Livingston, 2017).

Like multicultural and multiracial marriages, interfaith marriages are also increasing in the United States. Since 2010, 4 in 10, or 39%, married outside of their faith. This is in contrast to 19% in 1960. Interfaith relationships are even more prevalent today amongst unmarried people. Forty-nine percent are living with partners from a different faith. Jews, mainline Protestants and unaffiliated people are more likely to have interfaith relationships (Murphy, 2015).

There are several causes for the increase in the population of MII couples. One issue is immigration. The influx of Asians and Hispanics in the U.S. has created a larger pool of multicultural spouses in urban areas. Immigration from all over the world is increasing the number of MII relationships. Individuals have greater access to each other's culture. With the globalization of economy and education, people have been traveling outside their respective cultures at a faster pace. Air travel makes it easier to leave one's country. Another factor is the technological revolution of the last two decades. One can look on the internet and have direct access to diversity and heterogeneity. With a simple click, one can find out anything about a culture, society, race or religion. Even when looking for information pertaining to multicultural relationships one can find out what it's like, problems that occur and percentage of people involved in such arrangements. Individuals can find pictures and descriptions of where the other person has lived. He or she can even find out the origin of another person's surname. Thus, as soon as individuals meet, there is a certain level of familiarity that is already established. Google and other search engines make familiarity possible by showing individuals another person's home, haunts and lifestyles. People from foreign places are not so foreign anymore because the internet and social media can make them feel like they know each other. However, it can also give people an illusion of familiarity. People who are drawn to the otherness of the exotic or the marginalized, or the romanticized, may get just enough data to be seduced by the fantasy of finding themselves with the other. Unfortunately though, psychological differences and familiarities cannot be deeply understood through a website. Essig (2012) states, "Psychoanalytic meanings are found in the functional consequence of information, not in its abstract measurement. When it comes to the richness of experience, bandwidth isn't everything" (p. 452).

With regard to religion, individuals are becoming less religious and more spiritual. According to a September 6, 2017, report from the Pew Research Center (Lipka & Gecewicz, 2017), 27% of U.S. adults see themselves as spiritual and not religious. This increase is spread broadly over various groups: effecting African Americans, whites, Hispanics and people of varying education levels and party affiliations. If one is spiritual instead of religious there is a loosening of boundaries that makes it easier for people of different faiths to come together.

Another factor is the change in the legal and social barriers of the U.S. Since the Loving vs. Virginia 1967 Supreme Court decision, which struck down laws banning interracial marriage, it has become less dangerous in many communities to marry outside of one's race. The Obergefell vs. Hodges 2015 Supreme Court decision recognizing same-sex marriage has extended these laws to the LGBTQ population, further bringing people who are from different backgrounds together. In addition, according to current data (Balzarini et al., 2017) about 4%–5% of the U.S. population is involved in "consensually non-monogamous relationships". These relationships include those that are polyamorous. In many circles, boundaries in general, such as racial, cultural, religious and gender, are becoming more relaxed and fluid in the U.S. All of these factors contribute to the increased frequency of MII relationships. With these increased numbers, couples therapists must pay attention to the particular issues affecting these individuals.

We all have complicated internal lives that draw us to our significant others. Mitchell (2002) states that repressed wounds from early developmental phases tend to be reenacted with a loved one during adulthood. Intimacy implies that partners share warmth, trust, affection and cohesiveness. Erik Erikson (1950b) described the period between 19 and 25 as Intimacy vs. Isolation. It is the period when one hopefully develops the capacity to have a close relationship with another individual that involves trust, autonomy, and physical and psychological closeness. What causes people to be attracted to each other has to do with many factors, such as, biology, sociocultural issues, attachment styles, early object relations, as well as the replay of past psychological events between the couple.

Expanding on Bowlby and Ainsworth's attachment literature, Hazen and Shaver (1987) conceptualized attachment processes as a 'biosocial process' whereby affectionate bonds are formed between adult lovers. These bonds are informed by early attachment experiences from infancy. The three major styles of attachment that they delineated were "secure, avoidant and anxious ambivalent". They describe romantic love as a biological process that predisposes parenting in order to prevent species extinction. Moving through particular developmental stages such as romance and child-rearing can activate the early attachment system. Hazen and Shaver (1987) state that adult love is more complex than infant-caretaker attachment, although there are fundamental similarities. Psychosocial issues such as early loss, trauma, immigration, racism, anti-Semitism, parental divorce and academic performance affect partner selection, romantic experience and attachment experience in adulthood.

Scharff and Scharff (2014) conceive of romantic relationships using an object relations approach by expanding on Fairbairn, Klein, Winnicott, Bion and Dick's work. Object relations theorists begin with the premise that individuals are object seeking. Klein (1946) first came up with the term projective identification, whereby unwanted parts of the self are projected into another person. I see this concept as being key in understanding the relational dynamics in MII couples. Dicks (1967) felt that marriage was a continuous interaction of conscious needs, unconscious assumptions and working agreements. Bion (1967) described an ongoing feedback loop of projection and introjection that forms unconscious communication in infancy, between mother and child. I see this occurring all the time between MII couples. Scharff and Scharff (2014) extend these theories by perceiving couples as becoming "each others' internal objects, drawing from internal object relationships that preceded their finding each other and modifying them in the light of new experience so as to build new internal organizations" (p. 9). Shi and Scharff (2011) state that this process of "affective unconscious communication" is directly related to, and determines the quality of, long-term adult relationships. In addition, neurobiological factors have a profound effect on relationships between couples. Fishbane (2015) describes "the vulnerability cycle" (p. 691), when vulnerabilities are triggered in the limbic system if the brain senses a threat. Because the amygdala holds emotional memories from childhood, wounds from childhood can be triggered (by evoking emotional memories) by painful interactions between individuals. Romance causes individuals to have an interlinking psychic structure. MII couples share many commonalities in their romantic relationships, but what makes these relationships particularly complex is that they are also each drawn to the other by pre-existing and longstanding feelings of otherness (setting off a "vulnerability cycle" in their limbic system), albeit often in very different contexts.

Otherness dynamics in multicultural couples

Despite the fact that many MII couples are different culturally, racially or religiously, I find that many also have psychic homes that are similar. Individuals fall in love with each other because of particular commonalities. They might have grown up in a similar socioeconomic class. They might enjoy the same music or share the same ideals or culture. They might have a similar educational background. Mitchell (2002) states,

> It is difficult for me to imagine a person – or a human culture, for that matter – who doesn't orient himself around some sense of home: my place, where I am from, where I belong, where I long to return. . . . We seek continuity, sameness, as a way of grounding, anchoring ourselves, and each of us has our own particular way of going about establishing 'home'.
>
> (p. 36)

I believe that when one doesn't feel like he or she has a home, another person with similar, or familiar psychic struggles becomes the anchor. One is attracted in this case because the other person provides the possibility of finding home. What is not consciously realized is that it may be the other person's similar sense of lacking a home that is drawing the two together. The couple is (often unconsciously) banking on each one's otherness experience to generate togetherness.

When I speak to MII couples the key element I observe is that many have the psychic experience of feeling like the other or an outsider in their own culture, religion, race, community, peer group or family. This feeling of being an outsider often triggers a dissociated self state in one or both individuals. Bromberg (2011) states, "Defensive dissociation shows its signature through disconnecting the mind from its capacity to perceive that which feels too much for selfhood to bear" (p. 50). Self-experience occurs in unlinked self states that make a coherent whole personality (Bromberg, 1996). However, feelings of otherness, isolation and shame are often not integrated in one's psyche. Such individuals can, therefore, easily project their unintegrated feelings of otherness onto another individual who is recognized by society as (and is more visibly) the other. In an MII couple this 'other' individual is the spouse or partner.

With an interracial couple, each person's individual psychic experience is colored by their experience of their race. For example, if one is black, living in a predominantly white world, he or she will experience racism, social marginalization, oppression and inequality in every part of society. This originates in our history of slavery. These experiences are traumatic and affect the level of trust and safety that one feels in all aspects of life, both psychologically and physically. Racial prejudice and bigotry elicit feelings of otherness in non-white people. Other psychological events and traumas in these individuals' lives are also complicated and accentuated by the experience of racial inequality. Not only does one experience the pain of life's challenges, but also the pain of powerlessness, oppression, inequality and social injustice. This has a monumental impact on non-white people who live in the U.S.

In this culture, being white historically gives one a privileged existence in the community and overall social structure. This privilege creates a level of comfort as a social and cultural inhabitant. However, within that privileged existence, there are individuals who can experience themselves, for various personal reasons, as outsiders. So what might be the otherness that is felt in someone from the white majority culture? He or she might have experienced psychic marginalization or traumatic events in other parts of his or her life. Addison and Thomas (2009) state, "It is possible to be simultaneously privileged on some dimensions of identity and oppressed on others" (p. 21). Perhaps it was being an outsider in one's own family, school or community. Or maybe he or she felt that she never belonged in her peer group. Sometimes one has experienced sexual, physical or emotional abuse; bullying, drug or alcoholism; mental illness in a parent or sibling; or religious persecution (e.g. Islamophobia) in the community. This can cause him or her to feel like a psychic outsider. The otherness in this person is not necessarily visible. It can remain hidden because many of these issues elicit feelings of shame in an individual. The otherness experience of someone from a privileged majority culture cannot be compared to racism in a society founded on a history of slavery of Africans and genocide of Native Americans. And yet there is a shared feeling in an MII couple. Although racial issues mark a monumental difference in the life of each person, *psychic outsiderness or otherness is a shared intrapsychic feeling*. In other words, the common thread between these two individuals is this feeling of psychic otherness. Experiences of otherness, which may or may not be dissociated, draw people together. The feeling of not fitting in has a large impact on one's psyche. This often becomes a determinant of object choice. In MII couples, I have found that a major theme that reveals itself in the couples work is the conflict between belonging and otherness. The person who is obviously marginalized is not the only outsider in the relationship. Both may start out as outsiders in their own psychic way, when they find each other. They give each other a feeling of belonging, however, when a rupture happens in the relationship they return to a state of otherness, which causes both loneliness and isolation. How does this happen?

In the book *Loving: Interracial Intimacy in America and the Threat to White Supremacy*, Cashin (2017) describes the white experience of being in an intimate relationship with a person of color, particularly a black person. She states, a white person "can lose the luxury of racial blindness. . . . They can lose their blindness and gain something tragic, yet real – the ability to see racism clearly and weep for a loved one and a country that suffers because of it" (p. 5). Although, a black person is indeed perceived as 'the other', through social marginalization and racism, the white partner identifies with this otherness because of his or her own feelings of loneliness, isolation or guilt. In the couples work, the white partner may dissociate from his or her own feelings and focus on the otherness of his or her black partner. When disruption occurs in the relationship, what frequently happens when the therapist is white is that the couples therapist and partner from the majority culture can collude in focusing on the otherness as it relates to the person of color. On the one hand it is necessary to take the racism against the non-white individual into account. On the other hand, *the otherness experienced by that person has been internalized by the white partner, along with his or her own feelings of isolation.* This internalized, but dissociated, experience of otherness (in the majority/privileged partner) is often missed by the therapist. The outcome of this dynamic is that both individuals feel isolated and become outsiders (to each other) in their own relationship. In other words each person goes to their own defensive stance, where they are outsiders. The very issue that originally brought these people together now tears them apart. The outsiderness that now invades the relational field is further confirmed, and reinforced, by family, society and culture. The relationship that started as an antidote to this feeling of being a psychic outsider now reinforces each individual's feelings of isolation and loneliness. The experience of otherness that had been empathically internalized by the majority/privileged partner now gets extruded, projected out, externalized into the relational field and sits there like a wall obstructing intimacy, and possibly even generating self-doubt. Once the couple become derailed in this way, they are unmoored, with each floating in their own life rafts in the turbulent waters of their separate isolation. And the therapist can contribute to this by ignoring the shared psychic otherness in both individuals. The race/culture/ethnicity of the therapist may play a significant role in the selective inattention of the therapist.

Clinical vignette: I

An interracial couple came in to see me because they were arguing about 'little things' and over time felt "more and more alienated" from each other. Jane was 36, white, Scottish American and Christian. She was a teacher who grew up in an affluent suburb of NYC. Jamal was 38, African American and Christian. He worked as a physical therapist and grew up in a blue-collar suburb of NYC. The couple met at an Ivy League college 17 years earlier and had two daughters, aged 5 and 7. The relationship started out with both 'on cloud 9'. They shared the same politics and ideas about the world, and both volunteered for the same social justice causes. Both also felt different from their peers. As young children, they were both 'highly academic' and dreamed of going to Ivy League schools. Jane had a sister who had severe learning disabilities and suffered from OCD. Because of her guilt about being the successful child, Jane always kept her own intellectual successes from the family. Her parents were constantly focused on her sister, and Jane had to fend for herself. In Jamal's family, he was the first to go to college. It meant a lot to them because they were from a working class background. In the second meeting, when I brought up possible feelings of outsiderness for Jamal, both in his family of origin and the greater society, and for Jane, in her family of origin, they agreed. They both described themselves as never exactly fitting in, in their respective environments. It was initially surprising for Jamal to hear how much Jane felt like an outsider, because of his awareness of her privileged and affluent upbringing. However within her family of origin, she had always felt that she didn't belong. She grew up lonely and guilty for her success in comparison to her sister. Jamal, as a black man, experienced racism at every level. For example, even though he got straight A's, was an athlete and participated in student government, many people assumed that he got into college because of affirmative action. This and other macro and micro-aggressions made Jamal angry and heartbroken. Things were more difficult for him to achieve in society. He also felt guilt about being more successful than some of his relatives, who were traumatized by years of racism and poverty. Jane and Jamal were consciously attracted to each other for their independence and uniqueness, but *unconsciously* drawn together by their psychic otherness. However, the problems in their relationship started when they had children. With full-time jobs, they had less time for each other and became focused on the children's needs. Family members were also unhelpful, they felt, because they had less 'in common' with the other spouse's family. When their younger daughter started having some developmental issues, they found themselves adopting different ways of addressing the problems. Jamal felt that both he and Jane needed to sacrifice their very little personal time and help the child themselves. Jane wanted her daughter's school to take full responsibility. This put them at odds with each other. Jamal felt, as an African-American man, he could never really count on the help of government organizations, including the school. He also felt hostility from one of the white teachers, who acted as if he wanted 'a hand out' for his daughter. Jane's family of origin had access to lawyers and had successfully sued the board of education to get her sister into a private school for developmental disabilities. Thus Jane's view of what was possible was very different from Jamal's. Jane remembered that she always had to "stay under the radar" in her family because her sister's issues were so much bigger. She was afraid that her daughter was becoming like her sister. Jamal was afraid that if they didn't help their daughter, she would be left behind like those who couldn't succeed in his family. Thus for each one, but for different psychological reasons, the stakes around their daughter's difficulties were very high. The couple could not agree on the path to take with their daughter. Their daughter began to embody their racial split. Jamal, as a black man who experienced the intergenerational trauma of racism, felt mistrust toward society; Jane, in spite of her privileged position, was in touch with the otherness she felt as a child in her family of origin. Additionally, their biracial child had "the history of mixed race illegitimacy planted in her unconscious" (Bonovitz, 2009, p. 430). The systemic problems with their daughter caused each of them to become connected to their feelings of otherness, and to feel isolated and alone in their marital tensions. Jane felt overwhelmed by her daughter's problems, her own past of not belonging and the institutional racism that was experienced by Jamal and now their daughter. Jamal was overwhelmed by their daughter's problems, his sadness and anger regarding institutional racism and otherness, and his feelings that Jane, as his white wife, didn't understand.

The couples work focused on examining their feelings of estrangement, loneliness, racism, parenting, family of origin issues and communication patterns. A major theme of our work was addressing their mutual and projected feelings of otherness and helping them figure out how to help their children with school and issues around developing a biracial identity. When stress impacted the family system, the individuals returned to their independent mode, which was manifested by feelings of loneliness, isolation and otherness. It is important to look for aspects of otherness and split off self states in both members of the couple. This could bring forth feelings of connection that were lost over time. Bodnar (2004) states, "Dissociated self states lurk in social categories like a virus ready to erupt at the slightest stress to our systems" (p. 601). My experience with interracial couples is that each person has experienced feelings of being the outsider, and because this is a major theme in one's life, the relationship that once healed the sense of isolation can begin to proliferate the pain. This might happen more easily as time passes and other things besides the romantic relationship, such as work and children, become central to one's life. Cashin (2017) states, "The transition from blindness to seeing, from anxiety to familiarity that comes with intimate cross racial contact is a process of acquiring dexterity. And if one chooses to undertake the effort, the process is never-ending" (p. 5).

MII couples where one or both people are immigrants can also illustrate this point. The experience of immigration has its own set of psychological issues. Grinberg and Grinberg (1989) described the preponderance of mourning for immigrants who leave their country of origin. They mourn family members, friends, homes, community, sounds, smells and sense of cultural reality. There are complex ways that the human psyche accommodates to loss. Akhtar (1999, 2011) defines immigration as a third individuation. He states, "The separation-individuation phase contains elements of mourning because it leads to self and object differentiation. With each progressive move toward autonomy and identity consolidation there is an incremental loss of infantile omnipotence, symbiotic bliss and ego simplification through splitting and projection" (1999, p. 89). Rapprochement is integral to the process of differentiation. In multicultural relationships, all of these psychological processes are occurring alongside another person. Some individuals leave their country behind and decide to assimilate by marrying one who is from the host culture. This can be an unconscious means of feeling like an insider in a culture that feels impossible to navigate. It can also be a way of disconnecting from the pain of being an outsider, or a way to assimilate, globalize and integrate. But the conflict between the country of origin and the host country may be projected on to one's object choice (Akhtar, 1999). And those who marry outside of their culture might feel a sense of disenchantment with their family of origin, religious affiliation or community. Perhaps they break the boundaries of convention and live a life that is not defined by the status quo. Both partners live in a psychic home outside the mainstream. Otherness draws these individuals together.

Clinical vignette: 2

Catherine and Dinesh, an MII couple, met at their accounting jobs when they were in their mid-20s. Catherine was a 29-year-old white

Jewish woman who grew up in a Modern Orthodox family in a Westchester County suburb. She went to Jewish Day Schools but never felt like she fit into the system. She would question the existence of God, and when she was supposed to be at synagogue on Saturday, she would go to the mall with her secular friends from the neighborhood. All of her siblings were more religious. Her parents were frustrated with her because of her break from a long religious tradition. She always felt judged and traveled through life feeling like an outsider. Dinesh, a 30-year-old Indian American man, moved to the U.S. when he was 15. His father, who was a doctor in India, became a taxi driver while trying to take the "foreign medical exam". His mother worked in a retail store. The family fell on hard times when Dinesh's father had a car accident and had to be hospitalized for one month. He became disabled and gave up the dream of becoming a doctor. At 16, Dinesh had to start working at a law office to help support the family. He always felt like an outsider in the U.S. He was not like many in his Indian peer group, who came to the U.S. with money and status. He grew up Hindu and went to a private school while in India, which was run by Christians. Initially, he longed to return to India, where he had friends, a house and a life surrounded by family. As time passed, Dinesh assimilated by breaking ties with his Indian culture. He had no interest in an arranged marriage and only wanted to date white American women. In this way, both he and Catherine were outsiders in their family of origin and felt drawn to each other because of these differences. When the couple met at work, they felt as if they had "found their other half". They were close friends for about six months, began dating and married two years later. Catherine became enamored with Indian culture and felt saddened by the losses that Dinesh experienced as an immigrant. Instead of focusing on her own disconnection from her family, she felt deep sorrow for Dinesh, whose displacement was more obvious and visible. She began cooking Indian food and listening to Indian music. Dinesh felt that with an American wife, he could finally be integrated into American culture. After 9/11, the couple experienced blatant racism. Dinesh, who had brown skin, was called a terrorist when they were walking down a street in Manhattan. One evening some white adolescent men threatened to beat him up for being "Osama". These episodes were happening frequently in New York City and around the country. Catherine, who experienced white privilege, internalized Dinesh's brown skin. She felt the pain that the racists inflicted on her husband. Both Catherine and Dinesh felt marginalized but still had a sense of safety with each other. As the years passed, they began to have great success in their careers. They began coming home later into the evening and lost contact with each other. They stopped having sex. Catherine wanted to start a family but was confused whether Dinesh would be the right partner because their marriage felt 'dead'. As they saw each other less, they had trouble finding common ground. Dinesh had begun to feel more like an outsider in the U.S. Although he was a citizen, he was often treated like he didn't belong. Catherine was feeling his sense of being an outsider, her sense of being an outsider as a MII couple and her own sense of feeling like an outsider in her family of origin. They began drifting apart and questioning their own identities. What first drew them close now became an obstacle in their relationship. Dinesh started idealizing his early life in India. He projected his disappointment with his status in the U.S. onto Catherine. Although he had no intention of leaving, Catherine became obsessed with the fear of him leaving her to return to India. They loved each other deeply but felt lonely and lost in their identity confusion. They kept arguing about their loneliness and sought treatment to decide whether they should stay together and have children.

Catherine and Dinesh both felt like outsiders. Dinesh's feelings of alienation got more intense because of the bigotry that he faced in the U.S. Catherine was dissociated from her alienation from her family of origin and projected her feelings of otherness on to Dinesh. Initially when they were able to share their feelings of otherness, they felt less lonely and more cohesive. Now that troubles were occurring between them, they fell back into states of disconnection and dissociation. This became a rupture in their relationship and brought them to couple therapy. Throughout our work together, my emphasis was on exploring the interplay between racial prejudice and bigotry, projections and individual feelings of alienation and otherness. Catherine needed to disentangle her own feelings of not belonging from her empathy for Dinesh's more obvious and visible outsiderness. Dinesh needed to untangle his *need* for Catherine to be white and American (representing the prejudiced other) from his *desire* for her to be white and American (representing his own separateness from Indian culture). Attachment could only be reestablished when they could return to the otherness they shared rather than the otherness that divided them.

Intimacy is complicated, particularly for those who share differences that can't be denied. An immigrant's disappointment and anger with his or her host country, or country of origin, can be projected on to the spouse. This anger causes the spouse to get in touch with his or her own feelings of alienation and otherness, which has its origins in early life. The immigrant becomes a representation of the family that alienated the spouse in his or her childhood. Now, both members of the couple feel like outsiders. Attachment is disrupted. Alienation and loneliness ensue and cause marital strife.

Clinical vignette: 3

An interfaith lesbian couple came for a consultation because they were having problems deciding whether to circumcise their newborn son. Victoria, a 34-year-old, white Irish Catholic woman and Lena, a 33-year-old, white Jewish woman, had been together for six years. Victoria, a gynecologist, and Lena, a mental health counselor, complained about feeling a great deal of anger toward one another. They decided to come to couple therapy after a fight when Lena left the house and slept at a friend's house for two days.

Victoria grew up in an Irish Catholic household in New Jersey. She had three brothers and two sisters. All of them attended Catholic school and were baptized and confirmed. One of her brothers was a priest. Her memories of childhood and adolescence were steeped in Catholic experience and tradition. Life seemed positive and uncomplicated until Victoria reached early adolescence. Then with the awakening of her sexuality and her intense and persistent interest in girls she realized that she was a lesbian. Fearing that she would be discovered, Victoria became withdrawn, marginalized and sought out new friends and communities for support. Regarding religion, Victoria viewed herself as spiritual but was highly critical of the Catholic Church because of its stance toward abortion and homosexuality. She struggled with feelings of alienation until she became more involved in the gay community. Victoria met Lena when they were both working in the emergency room at a local hospital.

Lena grew up in a Jewish household. Her mother worked part time as an administrative assistant, and her father was a lawyer. She had two siblings, a sister and a brother. Lena's parents were part of the conservative Jewish community and felt that it was crucial for their children to be observant and involved. When she was in fifth grade Lena began to experience her attraction to girls. Over the next seven years confusion about her sexual orientation yielded to certainty. By her senior year of high school, she knew that she was gay. Lena felt like an outsider both in her family and the conservative Jewish community, which instilled heterosexual values. Lena found solace with other gay women after she left home to attend college and graduate school.

When Victoria and Lena fell in love, they felt a familiarity and connection they had never experienced before. They had been marginalized as lesbians and were outsiders in their respective conservative upbringings. They both considered themselves spiritual but not religious. They became fascinated with each other's cultural and religious roots: Victoria as an Irish American and Lena as a Jewish American. There was much they saw as common between them, including their conscious awareness of the commonality of their otherness in their families and communities of origin. While coming from different religious backgrounds, they felt they could talk to each other more easily than they could to people in their own religious communities.

After being together for six years, with "lots of fun and happiness", they decided that they wanted to have a baby. Victoria picked an anonymous sperm donor and got pregnant quickly. After the first trimester she found out that she was having a boy. The couple was ecstatic, but a snag in the relationship emerged when they began talking about whether their son should be circumcised. Victoria felt that the ritual was barbaric. She saw no evidence that could convince her that it was any better for the child. Lena wanted their son to be circumcised like her brother and father. She felt that all of his Jewish forefathers had been circumcised and she didn't have the heart to "change the course of history". Victoria felt that Lena was overburdened with a tradition that was no longer significant. They tried to discuss this issue together but always ended up yelling at each other and feeling misunderstood. The circumcision discussion opened up issues such as baptism, confirmations, bar mitzvahs and Christmas trees. They became acutely aware of their differences. How were they going to handle these issues with their children? They had spoken in depth and seamlessly decided how they would mother their son or daughter. Religion never seemed important. Now, the tension caused them to drift apart and return to a feeling of alienation and otherness each had experienced earlier in their lives.

Walsh (2008) asserts that clinicians need to develop what she calls "spiritual pluralism" (p. 73), i.e. a respect for different spiritual beliefs and practices. In order to best help these women with their difficult decisions, it was important to explore their own spiritual journeys and what caused them to feel disconnected from their faith. Assuming that a large part was religious conservatism toward their sexual orientation, what else caused them to feel disconnected from their religious identity and what kept them feeling connected? How connected did they feel to their family of origin? And what was the genesis of their feeling of otherness? This involves a slow exploration of each person's faith and helping them to understand why they felt detached from, or antipathy toward, certain rituals. A mutual exploration of their experience as outsiders would help them to reconnect and make the right decisions going forward. Although Lena felt that circumcision was one important link to the Jewish culture she wanted to preserve, they discussed other ways that they could create a combined religious and cultural heritage. Ultimately the baby was not circumcised.

When I work with a couple, I combine systems and psychoanalytic thinking.

I am informed by the history of racial oppression and white privilege in the United States, religious migration, interpersonal theory, object relations, attachment theory and systems theory. With an individual, my main focus is to understand the particulars of that person's developmental and relational life, including what goes on in the transference. With a couple, I focus on how each person's expectations, projections or anxieties are affecting the other (Rubalcava & Waldman, 2004). With an MII couple, I look at any systemic issues that might be affecting them. What is the impact of intergenerational trauma resulting from various aspects of racism on the family of origin? What is the impact of social class on this couple? Are family members supportive or unsupportive? What is the extent of the loss that is occurring for each individual? For the immigrant, is it the loss of a home or loss of being a part of the majority culture? Killian (2002) discusses a couple feeling like they lost their heritage after being turned away by their family of origin. The question might be if they lost their heritage, when did it actually happen and why is the loss so acute right now? And in what context did each of them feel like an outsider? What defenses do they use to cope with this experience? And where are the happiness and the sorrow in the relationship?

In this chapter, I have described a particular dynamic that can occur with MII couples. It is important to note that the couples therapist must also focus on global issues that affect mainstream couples such as power dynamics, sexual incompatibility, secrets, parenting problems, family of origin issues, communication breakdown and financial issues. However, MII couples are often subject to racial prejudice, bigotry, oppression and feelings of loss and isolation. They can become estranged from family members. As a white therapist who is in a MII relationship, I often forget that I have to pay attention to my own privilege because of my own dissociative processes. The experience of forgetting is a function of embodying white privilege. These dynamics might elicit guilt when I am working with MII couples. At the same time, awareness of the privilege can easily obscure my own experiences of marginalization and bigotry as a Jewish girl growing up in a majority non-Jewish, white community. It is important to look at the guilt and pain that is present in the treatment room within the therapist, as well as between the couple. MII couples may be dissociated from their guilt or pain. But as a therapist, it is crucial to understand which one of us bears the guilt and pain at any given time. When a member of a couple sees the internal issues that his or her partner is struggling with, a deep sense of empathy can be shared. What are the issues that they are projecting on to the other? And what are the enactments being replayed between them and with me? Feeling like an outsider begins early in one's life and is deeply painful. It can inform one's life and particularly become a foundation for one's intimate relationships. If individuals can discuss these feelings and share their pain, projections and loneliness, together couples can heal the wounds of their existence and become a secure home for one another, one that protects them from both a divisive world and a dissociated psyche.

Chapter 6

Forty shades of gray in intimacy for Iranians

Siamak Movahedi

The pursuit of intimacy in interpersonal relationships appears to be a global preoccupation.[1] This interpersonal quest is paradoxical in the digital age, when computers, smartphones and other digital devices compete for our attention, and we see many couples who prefer to engage with their iPhones or iPods rather than with one another in public or private. Intimacy is an ambiguous and confusing concept, particularly when it comes to any cross-cultural discussion, because it takes on different shades within and between different cultures. The term 'intimacy' in the West implies a sense of openness and self-disclosure in interpersonal space, an authentic sharing of feelings and experiences with a partner who listens and responds empathically. However, Schaefer and Olson (1981) have proposed a more expansive view of intimacy. They present intimacy as a complex interpersonal concept that consists of multiple dimensions, such as *emotional intimacy* (feeling close, ability to share feelings and be supported without defensiveness); *social intimacy* (having common friends and social networks); *sexual intimacy* (sharing affection, touching, physical and sexual closeness); *intellectual intimacy* (sharing ideas about and experiences with life and work); and *recreational intimacy* (sharing experiences, common pastimes and involvement in activities).

Intimacy thus comes to characterize the quality of interpersonal relationship. It refers to the pattern of interaction and/or the individual's capacity to enter into some form of social encounter we would consider intimate. Insofar as intimacy defines a mode of relationship, the significance of the culture within which it unfolds cannot be overestimated. Even if we try to define intimacy as a symbolic expression of deep unconscious feelings, projections, or pattern of object relationship, the nature of inner struggles within interpersonal encounters, and their mode of expression, are dictated by the available cultural repertoires of the time. Therefore, in any discussion of intimacy, we must remain cognizant of the cultural and structural issues that may enhance or restrict intimate interpersonal relationships and influence forms of interpersonal encounters. Since openness and self-disclosure seem to constitute a major part of intimacy, the experience of self and its cognitive presentation for disclosure to the other is within the cultural domain.

In its original meaning, 'intimacy' described the most private and concealed state of one's being. The term comes from the Latin *intimus*, which means 'innermost', 'deepest' and 'profound'. Its contemporary shift from psychic intimacy to intersubjective relatedness, personal to interpersonal, and private self to public self reflects a fundamental change in the structure of society and social relationships, as well as in our conceptualization of the concepts of individual, self and the interpersonal (Levenson, 1974; McKnight & Movahedi, 2017). Thus, to speak of intimacy as an intrapsychic – rather than interpersonal – phenomenon that operates outside the cultural surround, as some analysts framed the concept at the 2017 IPA Congress on Intimacy, is a residue of the old psychoanalytic concept of the subject as a self-enclosed monad.

The experience of the depth of the conscious and unconscious sense of the self in relationship with the other may differentiate between intimacy and closeness. For Burch (2004), closeness is located at the conscious level, while intimacy originates from the unconscious. Thus intimacy plays a much more important role in the therapeutic process than closeness.[2]

Although the contemporary concept of intimacy is part of the therapeutic culture that is indebted to psychoanalytic emphasis on openness in the analytic relationship, it captures a fundamental human need for being seen, acknowledged and understood by the other.[3] There is, of course, a difference between the needs of the individual and the cultural pattern of their presentation, recognition or even construction.

Some researchers have argued that there is a difference between cultures with traditional gender-role differentiation, individualistic cultures and collectivistic cultures in terms of the need for intimacy or its pattern of expression. Intimacy is said to be more salient in individualistic cultures, with its greater degree of gender equality, than in collectivistic or traditional cultures, which adhere to rigid gender-role ideology (Adams, Anderson, & Adonu, 2004; Chen, 1995; Hsu, 1985; Gao, 1991; Goodwin & Lee, 1994; Marshall, 2008; Wheeler, Reis, & Bond, 1989).

Marshall (2008) has examined the relationship between intimacy and gender-role ideology, and between intimacy and individualistic and collectivistic tendencies among European Canadians and Chinese Canadians. Her data reveal that Chinese Canadians display lower levels of intimacy, as defined by relational self-disclosure relative to European Canadians. However, the differential level of intimacy between the two groups was related to their level of gender-role traditionalism, rather than to individualism or collectivism.[4]

In light of this perspective, I will attempt to place the concept of intimacy within the context of Iranian culture, which is highly complex and layered, with many shades of gray. Here, to avoid a false dichotomy between the individual and the public narratives of intimacy, love and emotional relationships, we should note that cultures offer a template for the construction of individual stories; they provide the language for the organization of one's ideas, wishes, feelings and memories (Lévi-Strauss, 1951). In other words, cultures provide the syntax for a 'discourse' for which the 'vocabulary' comes from the subject's biography. At the same time, literary texts, novels, folktales and artistic expressions that center on intimacy may represent symbolic solutions to real but unconsciously felt social and cultural problems. That is, cultural narratives for intimacy tend to speak to people's experiences, conflicts and struggles in their gendered interpersonal relationships.

In a recent work, Movahedi and Moshtagh (2018) undertook a psychoanalytic study of a selection of traditional Iranian folktales, some of which continue to haunt individuals' consciousness and structure their fantasies about intimacy and gendered object relationships.[5] The world view underlying Persian folktales articulates the cultural dimensions of intimacy between men and women. *Scheherazade's One Thousand and One Nights* (known to American audiences as *The Arabian Nights*) is an excellent example of the man's fear of intimacy. Contrary to literal or historical interpretation of *One Thousand and One Nights* on a manifest level, Movahedi and Moshtagh maintain that it represents one story told 1,000 times. And the plot of that one story is the cure/domestication of an insecure, paranoid and narcissistic man who cannot stay in a relationship with a woman for longer than one night and will discard her – metaphorically kill her – the next day in search of a new affair.

According to their analysis, a major genre of traditional Iranian folktales centers on a woman who conspires against her husband, her betrayal of him, and her extramarital affairs. Women come across as dangerous, unreliable and shrewd – and never as honest, pious or strait-laced. Men, in contrast, are depicted as naïve and subject to easy manipulation. Many of the wives in these stories have lovers and send their unsuspecting husbands on a wild goose chase so that they can be intimate with their lovers in the husband's absence. As another folkloric mode of cultural expression, films have become a major context for the representation of changes in intimacy and the relationship between men and women within marriage in Iran.

In recent studies, McKnight (2016) and McKnight and Movahedi (2017) analyzed a longitudinal sample of Ann Landers's columns over a period of almost 50 years to identify how Middle America's narratives of marriage, love and intimacy had undergone a transformation since the 1950s. We have no similar resource for charting how the concepts of love and intimacy have evolved in Iran, but from what we can surmise based on some isolated research, various newspaper columns and what we hear on the couch or in supervision, there has been a tremendous degree of change in people's conscious need for intimacy. In this paper, I will attempt to flesh out and examine patterns in interpersonal encounters that may qualify as a form of intimacy.

I should note at the outset that my observations may be biased in terms of my informants' education, socioeconomic status, psychological mindedness and fluency in the therapeutic discourse of intimacy. The latter caveat is particularly critical, given that when it comes to notions of intimacy, Iranian culture is highly layered. For instance, we may notice significant differences between older and younger generations and between working class, urban traditional middle class, urban educated and secular upper-middle class when it comes to any discussion of intimacy.

I will begin by noting that the word 'intimacy' has no direct equivalent in Farsi – and that the concept of intimacy from 100 years ago in the United States is different from our concept today. Concepts have lives, and they evolve; they also enjoy many complex cognitive and affective dimensions. Simple translation from one language to another tends to miss some of the more subtle nuances; typically, only the denotative meaning is translated. This does not, of course, imply that people in Iran do not seek or engage in emotionally close interpersonal communication with one another. To the contrary, the boundary between formal and informal relationships in Iran is quite permeable, and impersonal interactions tend easily to become intimate and personal.

In a recent informal exploratory survey of a group of psychologists and psychiatrists for the purpose of identifying an equivalent word in Farsi of the concept of intimacy, *samimiat* (sincerity) was the most cited. Related words were also suggested, such as *nazdiky* (closeness), *doosty* (friendship), *hamrazy* (secret keeping, confidante) and *khodemani* (familiar).

I do not believe that *samimiat* (sincerity) captures the core semantic and affective dimensions of the English word 'intimacy' as it is used today; instead, a combination of all of the words suggested would come close to describing this multidimensional concept. The interpersonal experience of intimacy, or the quest for such an experience, does exist in Iran, although we may not find a single word to articulate the emotional richness of the concept. Perhaps no single word can do the job in any language.

Emotional intimacy

The definition of intimacy as emotional closeness and a reciprocal pattern of self-disclosure refers primarily to emotional intimacy. Emotional intimacy, ideally, is the mutual sharing of one's inner self, thoughts, feelings and fantasies. Intimacy and closeness are not necessarily related to love or sex, although people who are in love may feel very close and intimate without necessarily disclosing the depth of their souls to one another. Listen to this Iranian woman talking about her partner:

> I love him, he is a good man, he is not mean, but I don't have any feelings for him. He is uninteresting, kind of a retard; today I tried to break him down, picked on all his weak points, and tried to destroy him.

Another more extreme case is that of an educated professional Iranian man who claims to love his wife, but not to trust her with critical decisions. He disclosed that in his healthcare proxy, he put a friend in charge of life-and-death decisions rather than his wife. He said that at his deathbed, he did not trust her to participate in decision-making that would compel him to either receive or decline life-sustaining treatments.

The major complaint we hear today in clinical work with middle-class Iranian women concerns the lack of intimacy in their marital relationship.[6] The husband does not fulfill the wife's emotional needs: he is too busy with his work, too involved with his own family, and too absorbed by his own pursuits to listen to her concerns. There is usually a distant character in the past for whom they had a great deal of romantic feeling, but the real or fantasy relationship didn't go anywhere because of the differential social status of their families – the man's family wasn't good enough, he didn't have an advanced college degree, he didn't have a good enough job, prestige, title, or money.

Yet some Iranian women who married the man they fell in love with complain that after getting married they lost the sense of emotional intimacy with their husband, although they continued to get to know each other better. Something happens soon after marriage that causes emotional intimacy with their husbands to fade, although they may continue to have some level of *social, sexual, intellectual* and *recreational intimacy*. There is something in the gender-role-ideology of the marital relations that is hazardous to intimacy. The institutional structure of marriage, which favors male dominance, imposes a new set of boundaries that redefine the nature of the relationship that brought them together.

An astute woman observer recently commented at a focus group run by Moshtagh (2017):

> In this culture we don't own our body, especially our genitalia. . . . The ownership of our mind is not an issue. . . [it is] our vagina, [which] is a common property before the marriage, [but] becomes the man's property after marriage. That is enough to kill your desire, sense of agency, and any feelings of intimacy in the relationship.

This statement is of great significance for our discussion of intimacy. If a woman does not own the most private and intimate parts of her body in marriage, no sexual or physical intimacy with their legal owner will be possible: one cannot share with another what one does not own. This may be one reason for the flight into extramarital relationships in pursuit of intimacy.

Here we should note that equality and mutuality in relationships is the most important prerequisite of intimacy. Institutional gender inequality in marriage renders the potential for intimacy and its maintenance problematic. Iran's traditional gender-role ideology complicates the pattern of emotional intimacy, in terms of equality and reciprocity of self-disclosure. Self-disclosure is perceived as weakness and feminine, and the man – supposedly the dominant and more powerful partner – should not disclose the self to the woman, particularly since she is assumed to not be able to keep a secret.[7]

In the case of educated couples who either chose one another or were allowed to go through some type of courtship, albeit short, the experience of "the pure relationship", as postulated by Giddens (1992), may apply only to that short interval. The formal marriage seems to transform the pure relationship into mere gender roles. Some psychoanalytically minded women tell me that the nature of transference and countertransference feelings – in a generic sense – seems to undergo metamorphosis after marriage. One woman said:

> Before we got married, my image of myself and the image of me that I could see in his gaze were similar. After marriage, I became his contemptuous mother. His description and characterization of me had nothing to do with what I know about myself.

The objective reality of marriage had changed the subjective interpretations of the couple's identity in relation to one another: they could no longer recognize themselves in one another's marital narratives.

Today we can observe a profound change taking place in the nature of interpersonal relationships between men and women within and outside of marriage in Iran. This dramatic change has created what Durkheim (1893, 1897) called a state of *anomie* that has, in turn, created a cultural space in which a new form of intimacy between men and women can emerge. Because of this uncertainly in gender-role relationship, women are in a constant negotiation for their rights and privileges in marriage, while men continue to appeal to tradition to maintain their former prerogatives within the family structure. Yet, many men complain that women are castrating them and wonder what to do with their status loss. They report feeling emasculated at home and in the workplace.

This has created a crisis in the Iranian family and in heterosexual relationships, because engagement in deep and reciprocal emotional communication requires a relationship based on equality and mutual respect.

At the heart of any discourse of intimacy is the idea that individuals have emotional needs that require satisfaction, and that romantic partners should ideally provide that emotional satisfaction. The ideal of marriage is no longer one in which spouses simply fulfill their gendered roles, but also one in which two individuals satisfy each other's emotional needs within a context of mutual understanding and equality of attention (McKnight & Movahedi, 2017).

There is no intimacy in a master and slave relationship. This is why an increasing number of young educated Iranian women either do not marry or, shortly after marriage, file for divorce. Iranian newspapers even write about 'divorce parties' as an emerging fashion in some circles in Tehran (Bengali & Mostaghim, 2016). According to official estimates, more than 3 million college-educated Iranian women over 30 are unmarried. As one Iranian sociologist described the situation, "It used to be that a woman would marry and she would just have to get along. Now if she's not happy, she'll separate. It's not taboo" (Dehghanpisheh, 2014).

Women have surpassed men in terms of psychological, social, cultural and educational achievements. They are much more liberated, progressive and independent than men; a common complaint is that men are not educated enough, culturally free enough or socially sophisticated enough to tolerate living with a liberated woman. Today more than 60% of university students in Iran are women, and, equipped with degrees, many of them land good jobs. Their problem then is to find a man who is willing to marry a woman who is more educated and successful than him; this is one reason for a precipitous decline in the marriage rate and corresponding surge in the divorce rate.

Iranian women complain that their men may look fashionable and dress in designer suits, but mentally they are old-fashioned. Even highly educated Iranian men with advanced graduate or doctoral degrees, they argue, tend to hold regressive sex-role ideology and don't know how to behave toward women (Bengali & Mostaghim, 2016).

I have worked clinically with many highly educated Iranian couples in Boston. Some young men tend to act open-minded and liberal while dating a woman, but after marriage they become quite traditional and try to control the wife's work, dress and professional network of friends or colleagues. As a result, many such marriages soon fall apart. As one woman reports, "You can't marry a normal Iranian man who will not limit you and say, 'Don't work; don't go out'. These days it is difficult to find a really open-minded Iranian man. They are lagging behind us". Two women psychiatrists admitted that early in their marriages, they encountered great problems when their husbands asked that they not see male patients. One husband, himself a physician, had protested that he did not want his wife to listen to male patients' sexual fantasies.

Here I should note that contrary to the Western distorted image of gender relations in Iran, Iranian women are by no means losing the battle in their power struggle with men or even with the patriarch theocracy. They do not play a submissive and dependent role in marriage or in society. In fact women have been in the forefront of political resistance and responsible for much of the political, cultural and social change. They control a great deal of the contemporary social and political discourse.

In her recent travels to Iran, the Amsterdam-based photographer Marinka Masséus took a series of photographs of Iranian women defiantly throwing their veils in the air. These independent modern Iranian women, who were challenging the oppressive patriarchal system, impressed her immensely. The women she met told her they had two faces: "One for the outside world to stay safe and one for inside" (Elston, 2018). It is the inside face, of course, that is in search of an authentic sharing of feelings and experiences with a partner who listens and responds empathically.

Recently Dr. S., an analysand of mine who is a professor of surgery at a local medical school, was informed that hackers had broken into the university's human resources database and obtained vital personal data. She had to contact banks, credit companies, police and other agencies to inform them of the breach and to change numerous accounts to protect herself against identity theft. Despite the boring, bureaucratic and time-consuming steps required to protect her identity from being misused, she confessed that she was enjoying the whole experience. She had begun questioning who she was and which identity had been stolen. Who had been pretending to be her, and who was the real S.? Who was the real one and who was the fake one, and how could she be sure of that? At times the preoccupation sounded bizarre, as if she were struggling with identity loss, but the feeling was much more profound than pathological. She said that the feeling was similar to a person who had been imprisoned on a big farmhouse with many rooms and many trees. But then she had suddenly discovered a door to the outside, and she could see, through the opening, a vast vista of rich and pleasant new experiences. She said that she had been questioning her own identity: Who is this S., and whose identity has been stolen? Is she a human or a bird? She said:

> It didn't matter if I were a bird flying here and there. Was I a professor and a surgeon? It didn't, again, matter. I worked all my life to study, do research, write, and work to get this position, but now I felt it really didn't matter if I let go of it. So what was it that made a difference and could not be stolen from me? I felt it was love that made a difference; I could not do without [a] relationship with my sister, with my children, with parents, and with my patients in the ICU.

I was expecting to hear many other relationships that she had talked about in her analysis, when she said, "I feel comfortable to name people with whom I can let go of myself; I won't have to pretend or play a role. . . . I feel safe to be vulnerable".

It is interesting to note that the network of intimate relations in which Dr. S. can feel comfortable, can feel both safe and vulnerable – that is, the relationships in which she can be herself and not have to pretend or play a role – includes her patients in the ICU, but not her husband. In line with observations in other traditional cultures (Dion & Dion, 1993; Hsu, 1985; Ting-Toomey, 1991), marital partners in Iran experience less intimacy, because many of their intimacy needs are satisfied through close family relationships.

Despite this, many couples need to control and hold each other tight as they try to change the other. The Persian cliché that is used to define love as an instance of "one soul in two bodies" breeds disaster; it is simply a recipe for a power struggle over whose soul gets to occupy both bodies. This is also the plight of couples who share a similar pathology and stay together as a desperate solution to their attachment disorders and separation difficulties.[8]

Sexual intimacy

Emotional intimacy is not necessarily the same as sexual intimacy; they may not even be related. Although Giddens (1992) contends that the transformation of intimacy in modern societies invites the exploration of body and sexual pleasure, it is possible to have emotionally intimate relationships without being sexual and sexual relationships without being intimate (Jamieson, 1998). This is particularly the case in traditional Iranian culture, where many men and women tried to keep sex at arm's length from intimate emotional relationships, or believed that love was above and beyond the bodily experience of sex. The woman of a traditional Iranian man's fantasies was virginal and asexual, and shared her purity with his mother.

Interestingly, a number of studies by Iranian women researchers on Iranian women's sexual satisfaction attempt to present a picture of asexual Iranian women. Their respondents systematically underplay the importance of sex in their relationships, and report that sex is something private and that one may not even know whether she is satisfied with it. Many reportedly seek "serenity and support" rather than sexuality in their marital relationships. Some women report that they do not enjoy sex with their partners, and sex for them is a means of emotional connection. These are typical of women's responses:

> I am not young anymore, and my body's hormones work differently. When such serenity and support [can] be met by my husband, I have no conflict and this never bothers me. This is the condition which defines satisfaction for me.
>
> In a married life, it is not just a sexual relationship, it is living with another person who is with you every night and every day; you have such a relationship [sex] for just one hour.
>
> I think 10% of marital relationship is sex, but this 10% could complete the remaining 90%. In a common life, living issues capture 90% of our brain, and 10% of it is filled with sex. If you have good sex, just this 10% could solve many problems and other difficulties can be managed.
>
> Sexual satisfaction means one feels delight in everything and thinks nothing is better than this relationship. Then, she will bear all troubles. There will be a feeling of serenity and intimacy with her husband.
>
> Sexual satisfaction means just the feeling that my mind is free from problems, along with physical pleasure. If sex is based on principles, its pleasure is beyond any other pleasure; thus it can be defined as a pleasure from sexual tendencies besides mental serenity, and such sex is so rare.

In a qualitative study of women's sexuality in Iran, Farnam, Raisi, Janghorbani, and Merghati-Khoei (2016) reported that all the women in their sample engaged in sex with their partners primarily to achieve emotional intimacy rather than for the physical pleasure. They did not enjoy the physical part of sexual acts, although they admittedly enjoyed it only in condition of solitude through sexual fantasy and masturbation. Nobody in this study considered oral or anal sex as desirable, although some may have practiced it on rare occasions only to satisfy their husbands.

It is noteworthy that most of the studies conducted in Iran – and, paradoxically, by women – seem to give deference to traditional gender-role ideology and locate the root of marital discord and sexual dissatisfaction in economic factors (Darooneh, Ozgoly, Sheikhan, & Nasiri, 2017; Syasar & Bakhshani, 2014; Nasehi et al., 2017; Yekta, Raisi, Ebadi, & Shahvari, 2015).[9] Rather than a regressive sex-role ideology, economic conditions are blamed for problems with intimacy and sexual dissatisfaction. Demographic and economic, rather than cultural, factors account for sexual discontent. Studies report that women's sexual satisfaction is negatively correlated with their education – that is, the more educated the woman, the less satisfied she is in her sexual relationship with men. However, the relationship is reversed when it comes to the husband's education: The more educated the husband, the higher the wife's sexual satisfaction. This pattern is attributed, curiously, to income rather than to differential expectations mediated by education. Research findings also point to the negative relationship between sexual satisfaction and women's employment. That is, the professional presence of women in the economy is inversely related to their sexual satisfaction in marriage. This intriguing finding is also explained in terms of the stress women experience in working outside the home. There is no reference to education and occupation as factors that change the balance of power in a marital relationship and contribute to interpersonal discord. Rather than referring to women's increasing social and economic voice – and their subsequent reluctance to capitulate to repressive gender expectations – they name women's job-related stress as a factor in sexual dissatisfaction and marital discord.

We should, of course, be cognizant of the fact that these female researchers must be mindful of the gender-role ideology of the journal editors who will be vetting their papers, as well as the ideology of colleagues who will be considering them for merit or promotion. It is in that sense that they must begin their discussion by giving tribute to the constructive role of religious tradition in strengthening family life. From that perspective, sexuality is the path to motherhood, and the woman has no identity outside that position. In fact, we may argue that a major function of keeping the woman covered or out of sight is so that the man can maintain the illusion of separating from the mother, at least in visual fantasy. In some way, the best strategy for men (and also for women) to defend against Oedipal sexual feelings toward the mother is to deny sexuality in 'good' women (the mother) and restrict, punish or condemn any 'non-motherly' encounter with women who might arouse one's sexual desire. The justification for neutralizing the woman's sexuality is to get away, supposedly, from the abyss of sin and depravity. The underlying hope, however, is to turn the marriage into a simple asexual relationship of formal exchange and communication, and thus forestall the woman's sexual momentum or advancement. This is a major complaint we often hear in clinical work with women (Movahedi & Moshtagh, 2018).

The major part of sexual satisfaction in a marital relationship in Iran, according to the findings of these researchers, is fulfillment of the duties of a wife or husband. Women's contentment with their role performance in fulfilling their duties as a wife is the defining feature of their sexual lives. Yekta et al. (2015) report:

> Actually obtaining husband's love and his sexual satisfaction creates a sense of empowerment in women and are considered as values for women. A small number of women stated that they responded positively to their husbands' request *just for God's sake*. These women supposed themselves to adhere to religion, and were willing to do what great figures of Islam say about men and women's responsibility in marriage. Also, they had complete faith in compliance (Tamkin), which is emphasized in Islam.
>
> (p. 350)

A different study, by Khoei and Richters (2008), suggests that an idealized symbol of femininity for some Muslim Iranian women living in Australia is the notion of *tamkin*, or sexual obedience within marriage, by which the woman's modesty and self-respect is achieved by obedience to the sexual demands of the husband:

> By limiting sexuality to the reproductive period of life, Iranian women did not focus on sexual wellbeing in the broader sense as it might be understood

> by Australian women; instead, they regarded themselves as sexually healthy when no gynecological issues were experienced.
>
> (p. 191)

Khoei and Richters (2008) and Khoei et al. (2008) argue that the reason why Iranian women in Australia are reluctant to talk about sex with their internists or health workers is that Farsi lacks a vocabulary for inoffensive words for genitalia. In conversation with their children, Khoei and Richters report, parents coin their own words to refer to sexual organs. Here I should note that there are many Farsi words for genitalia, and their 'offensiveness' is not a property of the words themselves, but rather reflects the sociocultural attitude toward sexuality (Movahedi, 1996). However, the connotative dimensions of Farsi words for human sexual organs contain a great deal of aggression and belittling, and both men and women often use these words as expletives when cursing at one another.

Social intimacy

Contrary to the case in the United States, where Goldberg (1976) has argued that, as in the cliché, American men may have "many acquaintances but not one real friend", Iranian men form many close friendship bonds with their male friends. These friendships are not based merely on shared activity, but rather on a great deal of self-disclosure. Intimate friendships formed in youth extend through life and serve as the pillar of men's emotional relationships outside the family.

Examining Persian writings and literature, Kia (2016) argues that while an Enlightenment sense of self-other distinction defines Iranians' collective self, which is predicated on a mutually exclusive sense of difference, the modern Iranian self has been historically constructed through intimate friendships based on commonality and similarity. Men and women in Iran tend to form their own subcultures, within which they satisfy a major part of their need for intimacy.[10] Although they may be discussing the everyday details of life in their marital relationships, they tend to open their souls and disclose their secrets to friends or family members of the same gender.[11] That is, men and women tend to be more intimate with their same-sex friends than with their marital partners. While women are reluctant to disclose their sexual experiences to their male or female analysts, they tend to give detailed descriptions of their heterosexual encounters to close women friends. They share their private experiences with same-sex friends, even though they are also in competition with one another. In a series of focus groups that Moshtagh (2017) conducted at HamAva Psychotherapy Institute in Tehran, young women complained that they felt they were under scrutiny and negatively judged much more by women than by men. This was particularly true in reference to their mothers and fathers: "The one who would call you frivolous, empty, sloth, morally decadent [*kharaab*], and even whore [*jendeh*] is usually another woman". They felt that some form of primitive competition between the mother and daughter extends to relationships between women. A number of young women reported that they had to hide their achievements from their mothers, but not from their fathers. With their mothers, they could primarily share their agonies and failures; otherwise, the dynamic could become volatile. This experience, they felt, characterized the nature of their close relationships with women friends, in that they could share their grievances and worries with one another, but not their successes.[12]

Finally, exploration of the cultural modes of emotional connection is incomplete without a discussion of the ritualized management of failed intimacy. This is particularly relevant when a person does not want to break off a relationship, but instead seeks to negotiate a condition for its amelioration. Interpersonal management of the sense of having been hurt by the other party in an emotionally close relationship takes different passive and active forms. But the most salient form of an attempt to restore an intimate emotional state is through a ritual of distancing and symbolic communication in which one is not on speaking terms with the other person. This mode of reparation, called *ghahr* and *ashti* in Farsi, is part and parcel of every Iranian's repertoire for dealing with failed intimacy. *Ghahr* occurs within important affectionate relationships and is communicated through nonverbal codes signifying that the person has no desire to speak with the other. It is a ritual of total withdrawal from any interaction with the person, who has supposedly violated the code of mutual respect and empathy for the aggrieved party (Behzadi, 1994). A heightened degree of interpersonal sensitivity within Iranian culture, similar to what Roland (1988) labels 'radar-sensitive' in the context of Indian culture, is according to Behzadi, responsible for this ritual of disengagement-reengagement; here the role of the third party is critical in restoration of the failed intimacy. *Ghahr* is a communicative act that is addressed to the guilty party to elicit his or her feelings of guilt, shame, regret, love and compassion, and also to others so that they will intervene to mend the relationship and trigger a reconciliation process called *ashti*. *Ghahr* is thus a cultural ritual of reparation and reconstruction of failed intimacy. There is a popular Persian poem that may capture the spirit of this ritual of disengagement-reengagement:

> *I tear this thread between us,*
> *So that it would get shorter when we knot it back,*
> *drawing us closer than before the crack*
> (my translation)[13]

Notes

1 I wish to thank Gurmeet Kanwal and Salman Akhtar for inviting me to contribute to this valuable collection of papers. I particularly wish to thank Nahaleh Moshtagh who generously shared her thoughts with me on this topic and made many insightful comments and suggestions on earlier versions of this paper.

2 Burch (2004) observes that some people perceive angry relationships as a sign of being intimate. However, he sees merely intense engagement in such relationships without them being either close or intimate.

3 In his frequent advice to Martha, Freud (1961) emphasized that the key to emotional intimacy in their relationship is "absolute openness and truthfulness in your communication without holding back" (p. 266).
4 Here we should add that the "individualist" and "collectivist" cultural distinction is quite problematic and superficial; both concepts are multidimensional rather than linear. Yet according to the findings of a global survey, a mix of strong family ties and connections and a high degree of individualism characterizes Iranian culture (Javidan & Dastmalchian, 2003).
5 Such individuals have treated folktales as a cultural graveyard in which many of those invisible creatures reside. In that sense, every folktale is seen as being embodied by ghosts of the dead that continue to invade the present, and caution against any change in the future.
6 Recently a therapist who works in two different clinics in Tehran, one in the prosperous part of the city and the other in a poor part, reported that while in the well-to-do section of the city women's primary object of grievance is their husbands, she does not hear any talk about marital discord in the poor section of the city.
7 There is a cultural belief, as reflected in Persian proverbs, that a man should not trust a woman with any secret. "A woman does not let the pea wet in her mouth" (Zolfaghari, 2010, p. 1143); that is, "A woman conceals what she knows not" (Ardakani, Harehdasht, & Hajjari, 2015).
8 "Fusion and merging does not create intimacy, but an illusion of it"; "For the intimacy to happen[,] one has to be able to have sense of self; one needs to know one's own boundaries, as being enmeshed is not intimacy" (Purser, 2007, p. 296).
9 In a study of 532 young married women in Tabris, the researchers report that 66% of women were suffering from some form of sexual dysfunctions (Mohammad-Alizadeh-Charandabi, Mirghafourvan, Asghari-Jafarabadi, Tavananezhad, & Karkhaneh, 2014).
10 Sociologists have long argued that subcultures develop in response to group problems of adjustment, so that actors will be able to cope with their collectively experienced problems of adaptation. Downes (1966) posits that subcultures arise "where there exists ineffective interaction with one another, a number of actors with similar problems of adjustment for whom no effective solution as yet exists for a common, shared problem" (p. 7).
11 Here Burch's (2004) distinction between intimacy and closeness challenges our use of the term 'intimacy', in that many women have reported that they feel close to their same-sex friends without experiencing a deep sense of positive contact unconsciously. That is, their feeling of positive contact at a conscious level is not necessarily matched by a similar feeling at a deeper level.
12 A British sociologist, Winch (2013), has presented an interesting argument that the "girlfriend gaze" plays a much more important role in the construction of contemporary mainstream femininity than the male gaze. The culture of friendship among women is the most important source of their feminine identity.
13 *man reshteh y mohabbate tu pareh meekonam shayad gereh khorad, beto nazdeektar shavam* (Zoghi Ardestani, The Poet)

Chapter 7

Privacy and intimacy as two mediators of relatedness

Suzanne Benser

Bion (1962) and Winnicott (1971) brought to psychoanalysis the concepts of transitional space, containment, the drive to know and normal projective identification. These concepts have allowed psychoanalysts to recognize how internal and external realities become constructed developmentally and underlie internal representations of self and others. Those internal representations carry 'gradients' (Levy, 2017) of relatedness between self and others that are manifest in interpersonal relationships and the analytic relationship. The interplay of privacy and intimacy mediates those gradients through the subjective sense of self in relation to the sense of others.

This contribution begins with psychoanalytic perspectives on privacy, including the development of the ability to 'keep secrets' and the complementary role of the analyst's privacy and analytic reverie. Psychoanalytic perspectives on intimacy follow, with a consideration of the tension in the clinical setting between the analyst's privacy and disclosure. A detailed clinical illustration follows of a patient whose interpersonal oscillation between seductive and disappointing interactions with others was recognized in treatment as a compromise between narcissistically fused internal self and object relationships and a push towards greater self agency. The discussion and conclusion conceptualize the analyst's crucial use of privacy and intimacy in patients with difficulties in psychosexual development.

Theoretical perspectives

Privacy

The capacity for privacy is a component of the ability to recognize one's self as separate from others. It begins when children realize that they know things about themselves that others are not aware of and continues to develop as children learn to keep secrets. Greenacre (1960) noted that secrets could be used in ways similar to fetishes; they can bridge the gap between self and object, defend against separation anxiety, and ensure corporeal integrity. Margolis (1966) described how secret keeping further develops when children feel the strain of believing parents can read their disturbing thoughts. He delineated the conscious and unconscious aspects of keeping secrets and how shame and guilt experienced in object relations around sexual feelings and fantasies can lead to keeping secrets from one's self and others. Thus, secrets can be used as stepping stones in the development of independent thoughts on the way to developing the 'capacity to be alone' (Winnicott, 1958a). Gentile (2013) has written about ways in which 'secret keeping' becomes facilitated through games such as hide-and-seek and truth-or-dare.

Ogden (1991, 1996, 1997) has written extensively on the analyst's need for privacy and the essential contribution of analytic reverie to the analytic process. He defines personal isolation as a natural response, a "protection against the continuous strain that is an inescapable part of living in the unpredictable matrix of human object relations" (1991, p. 385). Cooper (2008) refers to the analyst's privacy as "a place for the analyst's self-reflective activity". In the contemporary model of analytic reverie, these views on analytic privacy have been incorporated with Bion's conceptions of 'suspension of memory and desire' (1970) and 'maternal reverie' (1962). These perspectives have integrated the reflective aspects of privacy and the containing function of reverie and led to recognition of the therapeutic aspects of the analytic third.

Intimacy

Intimacy has different connotations but is most commonly used to describe a 'gradient of relatedness' that includes a transcendent emotional experience associated with the disclosure and recognition of one's self. Levy (2017) described the analyst's ability to experience intimacy through openness to unconscious communication and connection with bodily experiences. In consonance with Bion and Ogden's theories, he views the analyst's capacity for intimacy as dependent on the resilience of his object relations: "Intimacy may be defined as the capacity to tolerate turbulence resulting from the object's presence, without autistically avoiding contact or omnipotently merging through projective and intrusive identifications" (p. 8). Kantrowitz (2009) writes about the tension in psychoanalysis between privacy and analysts' self-disclosure. She states that "there has always been a tension between privacy and self-disclosure in psychoanalysis. It has manifested itself differently over time, but concern about revealing too much or too little exists in every rendition of the analytic landscape" (p. 790).

The fundamental rule of free association was standard practice in the classic psychoanalytic tradition. With the goal of preventing the analyst from unduly influencing the patient, the patient was asked to forfeit privacy while attributing to the analyst the task of disclosing as little as possible. This perspective, with its underlying narrow conceptualization of transference/countertransference as fundamentally intrapsychic and devoid of interpersonal contributions, is now seen as excluding important aspects of the analytic relationship with therapeutic benefit. In contemporary theories, conscious and unconscious elements from both patient and analyst contribute to the uniqueness of the relationship that allows the patient to develop greater connection with his or her subjectivity.

The relational model views the analyst's abstinence as lacking in authenticity since nonverbal or unconscious aspects of the analyst contribution can be 'read' by the patient. Thus, Cooper (2014) acknowledges the impossibility of the analyst 'hiding' his/her subjectivity; he refers to such abstinence as an 'illusion of privacy'. Winnicott's (1958) contributions elaborate the paradoxical nature of privacy and intimacy that underlies the difficulty in defining an 'ideal' analytic stance: "The basis of the capacity to be alone is a paradox; it is the experience of being alone while someone else is present" (p. 417).

Post-Bionian writers refer to the entirety of the interactions between patient and analyst as the analytic field and consider mutual recognition as the therapeutic goal.

> The hypothesis we propose is that the (*analytic*) field is a conceptual tool that enables us to modulate in a fine-grained and safe manner the distance between patient and analyst, and to achieve and expand emotional unison – in our view the central therapeutic factor.
>
> (Civitarese & Ferro, 2015, p. 69, italics added)

The elaboration of concepts related to the analyst's capacity for intimacy and privacy laid the foundation for much of the growth in psychoanalytic theories. The interplay of privacy and intimacy needed for analytic reverie comes to the foreground of the analytic relationship when sexual desire is manifest. As Davies (2013) described in her follow-up to her now classic paper on erotic countertransference, "Love in the Afternoon": "We know from our own personal experiences that talking sex can be as exciting or even more exciting than doing sex" (p. 171).

Fonagy's (2008) conceptualization of sexual arousal as an experience that can betray the subjective sense of self-containment explains how sexualized patient material can become burdensome for the analyst when it 'bypasses awareness' and presents as unwelcome bodily arousal:

> It will always be an imposed burden . . . unless we find someone to share it with. What Freud (1905) talked about as an objectless state, and Laplanche (1995) and Stein (1998) as the 'enigmatic other,' we describe in terms of an alien part to the self internalized by the alienating parts of the mirroring object-mother. . . . This leads to the paradoxical and vacillating dimensions of shame and excitement in normal sexuality. The shame associated with the rejection from the Oedipal parent alternating with the non-contained erotic enigmatic experiences fuel that adult's sexual fantasies, and choice of love partners. Current experiences that activate the non-contained erotic experiences sometimes bypass awareness and 'burden' the self with unwelcome bodily arousal.
>
> (p. 23)

Thus, sexual feelings in the analytic relationship carry the oscillations of excitement and shame associated with usual Oedipal development and can be used to help mentalize the non-contained or alien aspects of psychosexuality. In patients whose intersubjective experiences have not allowed them to 'share' the imposed burden of sexuality in fantasies and in love, the excessiveness of sexuality is experienced as threatening to attachment and must be split off and projected. When the excessiveness is projected onto the analyst, it can become an unconscious communication that presents an additional burden for the analyst with unwelcome bodily arousal.

A detailed clinical illustration

Mr. A was a student in his mid-20s who had just started a graduate-level business program when he began treatment with me. He had struggled with anxiety, chronic insomnia and migraine headaches as a child, all of which had remitted somewhat in college and were now back worse than ever. He had additional physical symptoms, including neck pain with TMJ and a history of having broken his back in the first grade in a serious bicycle accident, followed by a two-year long convalescence. He had a world-weary demeanor that was at odds with his description of himself as anxious and hypochondriacal. I also found his presenting complaints incongruent with the revelation that he was quite athletic and had participated in a wide range of individual sports since he was a young child.

He described being very close with his mother and said, "She is fantastic, we are a lot alike, and honest with each other". During the first year of treatment he would ask her opinion about surprising things and follow her suggestions without question, only reporting these events in retrospect. He had multiple girlfriends throughout the country and spoke with his mother openly about all of those relationships, seemingly having no secrets from her. One of his "on again, off again" girlfriends lived in his nearby hometown and was 'good friends' with his mother. Both he and this girlfriend spoke with her about the details of their sexual relationship.

My internal response was concern for the lack of privacy with his mother. He said his mother could "read him like a book", but that others found him complicated. I wondered if the apparent narcissistic fusion with his mother had been longstanding, and to what extent it had precluded him from thinking his own thoughts and developing a defined sense of self and others.

Another presenting problem was that "he was sick of being pissed at his father". Mr. A described his father as absent and alcoholic and was deeply disappointed when he discovered the father had had a long-term affair with someone in the family circle. The parents had separated after the 'discovery' for nine months, and Mr. A voiced a wish that his mother would leave the marriage. Most poignantly, he described his own yearning for his father to recognize him. He related "begging his father to play catch with him" as a child and giving up on trying to bond with his father when he became aware of the affair.

We began working together three times a week and he moved to the couch after a few weeks. Mr. A brought in dreams frequently from the beginning of the three-year treatment. Since childhood, he had recurrent dreams involving car accidents that usually involved his father driving off a ledge, and with Mr. A observing, frozen in shock. He had a similar recurrent dream of himself driving a car with his mother as the passenger, also driving off a ledge. Another recurring theme was being in fights, often with guns involved, in all of which he was ineffectual in defending himself.

Our work began with exploring the experiences of danger and shock in his dreams. The references of falling off a ledge undoubtedly carried the trauma of the accident that left him bedridden at home for nearly two years with a broken back. I began to sense the fear of death mixed with desire that he experienced during that period of close confinement with his mother and sisters. The shock in seeing his father "driving off a ledge" seemed to convey the fear-wish of his ambivalent, dangerous feelings, wanting more closeness while hating his father for his absence, while also wanting mother to himself. I wondered if the dream of driving off a ledge with his mother was a wishful revision of his accident in which he was not alone as he had been in the original accident and would not be separated even as they fell to their death.

Other references to falling were in early memories of his eldest sister dropping him on his head mixed with a memory in which he pulled a younger baby sister off the television, preventing her from falling. I came to understand that he had felt deeply lonely as a child, despite his current conscious feeling of being close to his mother and several of his sisters. He had six siblings and at times felt himself as an outsider to the close-knit group of five sisters and mother. I wondered if the birth of his two-year younger sister left him abandoned, unsafe and unregulated. Not only had his father refused his bids for recognition, but he had also favored his only brother, who was three years younger and despised by the patient.

Mr. A's paradoxical self-representations as athletic and hypochondriacal gave way to frequently presenting himself as 'cocky' and self-confident, which was consistent with his habit of wearing form-fitting clothes that revealed his toned physique. Seeing himself as a perennial bachelor, he was clearly confident in his ability to attract men and women sexually but had been unable to feel a sense of sustained safety, connection or satisfaction in sexual relationships. I suspected the dreams with fights and guns referred to an internal sense of danger around sexuality, with the nature of the danger not yet apparent at this point in the treatment.

We began to explore his history of promiscuity that had begun from an early age. He often had had sex in his parent's home in high school, describing the experiences with a flat, empty tone. We established that he was unaware of any fear, or thrill, of being discovered. Since then, he had had relationships with several girlfriends with whom he had repeated cycles of yearning, disappointments and breakups, while simultaneously engaging in sex with nearly anonymous partners. He had had sex with a few men, some friends and others anonymous, and had found those encounters even less satisfying. He was deeply embarrassed when friends saw him with "anonymous women" and felt shame in being known as a 'player'.

Mr. A seemed to have a limited capacity to hold and process the excesses of desire through mental and physical actions. I understood his compulsive sexual activity as dissociated attempts to evacuate the overstimulation, shame and envy he had experienced in the mix of emotional neglect and overstimulation in his early object relations. I wondered if the yearning for his father had led to an identification with him as a philanderer, accompanied by the projection of envy of his siblings and father's lover onto his betrayed girlfriends. Insecurities around his physical self were likely linked to these attachment difficulties and compounded by the accident. In a possible condensation of his penis and broken back, he may have looked for reassurance of his bodily integrity through sexual activity. I hypothesized that the lack of integration of his bodily feelings with his object related experiences, and the use of objects for evacuation, left him vacillating between yearning for meaningful connection and feeling hollow and anxious.

Mr. A's increasing ability to verbalize a wide range of shameful and fearful subjective states, including those associated with his sexuality, led me to feel that I was reaching him. My recognition and linking of his affects with relational experiences seemed to be resonating with his burgeoning self-recognition. His dreams shifted from driving off mountains to mountains that might erupt, and when dreaming of fights, he could now defend himself with 'rubbery' arms. He was relieved that he felt a greater sense of agency in his dreams and a lessening of the anxiousness during the day. Another sign that Mr. A was developing increasing awareness of his internal state was his recognition that shameful feelings associated with his compulsive sexual activity were contributing to the oscillations in his experiences from cockiness to emptiness. He thought he might be able to "stop the cycle" if he "fell madly in love".

A shift occurred in Mr. A's previous generic descriptions of his girlfriends when he made an allusion to the lack of trustworthiness of several of his girlfriends, who he now described as having "seemed sweet but turned" on him. As he conveyed a conversation in which he had been discussing this with his mother, he described her as having faults for the first time. He said his mother was not supporting his choice of girlfriends and wanted him to "choose someone more adult, more like herself". In the session on the following day, he told me about an older woman professor who was teaching him a course, who he could tell, "wanted to get fucked". With an insinuating, caressing tone, he told me he "liked older women", and "they liked him", since he was in fifth grade. For the first time, I became fully conscious of his evacuating excessiveness into me, as I became simultaneously aroused and ashamed, the older woman whose secrets he knew.

The unbidden sexual feeling was an intrusion into my analytic privacy and brought with it the awareness that I had been suppressing a building erotic/shameful undertow. Mr. A had telescoped our generational difference by turning the teacher/analyst/mother into the one who was in need. I did not feel able to 'tolerate the turbulence resulting from the object's presence' (Levy, 2017) without projecting the mix of 'too-muchness' (Benjamin, 2015) and shame back at him from a position of judgment in which either he or I would be accused of seduction, either the 'doer or done to' (Benjamin, 2004). This led me to ask if his parents knew he had had sexual experiences with older women, realizing I was looking for someone to contain our experience along with my preconscious realization that the "older women who liked him since the fifth grade" were probably teachers who had sexually transgressed with him. Before attempting to address the transference/countertransference experience directly with Mr. A, I needed to re-establish my self-reflective capacity. Over the next several months I sought consultation with a colleague to further support my internal processing of the patient's material. During this period, Mr. A's dreams continued with the theme of heights, but shifted from mountains that might erupt to tall buildings actually exploding, including my office building. I recognized that he had projected his phallic narcissism onto me, and that our analytic field could not yet contain his explosive sexuality, shame, rage and envy.

Throughout the second year of treatment, we renegotiated the interplay of privacy and intimacy between us and found a better, and safer, distance from which to continue our work. He continued in the cycle of sexual acting out followed by periods of emptiness and desolation. He talked about knowing he could "get under people's skin" and "manipulate women" while "women were coming out of the woodwork", even as he "tried to break the pattern". My countertransference experiences indicated his mother likely projected her omnipotent sexual and shameful feelings into him as he had done to me, and perhaps as he had projected onto the teachers who had violated his boundaries. I remained quiet for much of the material and sensed the seductive undertow between us slowly remitting.

Mr. A began occasionally missing sessions, and in talking about those sessions, he began talking about his difficulties with time. He felt that time was slipping away and that he was 'the same' since he was 14 years old. I wondered if this was a traumatic re-experiencing of his convalescence, along with a manifestation of his difficulties in engaging more fully in the external reality of our relationship (Bach, 2006). It also seemed that he had brought in the emptiness he experienced after compulsive sexual activity, now projecting the experience of neglect onto me, rather than the earlier overstimulation and shame.

Mr. A made an uncharacteristic comment in a session during this period. He wondered if I remembered the end of a previous session. While recounting to him my recollection of the session and discussing the possible meaning for him of that experience, I became aware that he attributed something to himself that I had said. In that interaction, I recognized his attempt to hold in his mind both our subjectivities, that I could remember something he did not, as well as his bid for narcissistic fusion in coopting something from my mind. I wondered if he was becoming more able to tolerate the 'turbulence of my otherness' and persisted in bringing to his awareness the coopting of my words.

We were able to make connections between his feelings that women "can seem sweet but turn on you" with the feeling that his mother used him as a stand in for his absent father, as well as the older women who "turned on him" and used him sexually at a young age. I understood more fully his shame when friends saw him with another brief hookup; he felt this revealed the 'secret' of having been used by his mother and older women. He was able to maintain the restructuring of reality (Colarusso, 2009) in which the anonymous women were the shameful ones who were "coming out of the woodwork" and "wanted to get fucked", but he could not maintain that maladaptive defense when he was in a triadic position with his friends. He saw himself through their eyes, the shamed one who would have sex with anyone who was equally empty. I wondered if it also brought to his mind the split-off envy and betrayal by his father as he saw his own betrayal to his girlfriends through his friends' eyes.

He dreamt of a floating spaceship, where he lived with his family, a wife and son. They were going to "take over the world" and landed by his childhood home and "burned the hell out of everything". We heard how in the third grade, his mother gave him "the birds and bees talk, how babies were made", and how disillusioned he was the first time he had intercourse: "It was too easy, and it was supposed to be special". He was happy he could recapture the poignant belief that "it could be special" in the dream of having created a family.

Towards the end of the second year of treatment, Mr. A was absent for several sessions after a visit to his hometown. He was very apologetic about missing the sessions and said, "I hate it when others are irresponsible with me, and then I do it to them". He recounted feeling very defeated by his father's lack of recognition during the visit and angry that everything was "always on his father's terms". Over the course of our work he made fairly frequent references to literature, noting that he read extensively during his long convalescence. During the session in which he was apologetic for his absence, he said he "felt like Colin, the kid in the *Secret Garden* (Burnet, 1911), the one in the wheelchair in the garden".

The *Secret Garden* tells the story of young adolescents coming of age. Mary, a neglected, but spoiled girl, is transformed as she discovers the wonder of life and relationships. The beginning of her transformation is associated with her first real friendship, with a boy named Dickon who connects deeply with animals and all growing things, and they discover a magical garden that they keep secret. Mary then feels compassion for the first time, for another neglected but spoiled character, Colin, who has a psychosomatic back problem and is wheelchair-bound. Colin's father has shunned him because he reminded him of his mother who died in a tragic accident when Colin was very young. He 'spoils' Colin in ways that are always 'on his terms,' only giving him things that perpetuate his illness and dependence. Mary reveals to Colin the existence of their secret garden and makes repeated attempts to convince Colin the garden will cure him. His physical ailments are indeed cured in the garden, and the three of them eventually share magical and transformative experiences that deeply connect them with the aliveness in themselves and in their garden. I noted to Mr. A that, like Mary, I saw him as a potentially healthy young man whose father could not show him his love and affirm him because of his own difficulties.

A few months later, in a visit back to his hometown, Mr. A had a conversation with his father in which he felt he was open with him for the first time. He became aware that his resentment for his father had kept him from recognizing and expressing his underlying admiration for him. He told his father he thought he was a 'good man', and noted that he now felt relieved and less angry with his brother as well.

During a session when he seemed particularly empty, he recounted a 'joke' in which he called his girlfriend a slut, followed by noting the irony he perceived in the joke, since he was the "mother of all sexual indiscretion". It seemed he was now enacting a more elaborated fantasy that could further the containment of his degraded sexuality. The 'slut' girlfriend representation was more differentiated from the analyst/mother/teacher representation, and he was able to oscillate between self and object representations. In calling himself the "mother of all indiscretion" he assumed the parental position; he was the 'mother' who was indiscrete but able to use discretion/regulation, not the openly shamed, exposed and unregulated slut. Thus, he could not yet fully give up the omnipotent narcissist fusion to regulate the shame he associated with being overly stimulated.

Around this time, another shift occurred as he reported his mother being angry with him for the first time, saying his mother "was 'pissed' I didn't come home for a big family dinner". He went on to talk about realizing he could hurt his parents by moving away. This was the first time he recognized his mother as being affected by him as a separate person. The development of his ability to recognize and empathize with others as objects he could be angry with, and who could be angry with him, heralded the beginning of the remission of his emptiness and anxieties. The cycles remitted during the last year of treatment; he seemed more alive, and time was no longer "slipping away".

He began talking about moving from the area after graduation and ended treatment after deciding to move quite far away for a promising position. He wanted to "subsume himself in something bigger" and was "curious to see how I'll be on my own". He told me he had never been able to be his "natural self" with Dr. M, his previous psychiatrist who was also his parents' couples therapist, but that he had been with me. "I'm going to be OK on my own and I will get to see how much treatment has done". I also knew he was going to be OK on his own; he could now leave me behind as a separate person much older than he, to a world of peers, with whom he could experience the aliveness of their own secret garden.

Discussion

Mr. A had found a way of using his poignant sexual longings to attract others but had not been able to move forward in satisfying his yearning through mature sexual relationships. He had no way of 'using' the relationships with his parents to regulate his sexual feelings and the associated affects and rise to the demands of the sexual (Benjamin, 2015). From his first experiences with intercourse in high school, his sexual experiences were dissociated from psychologically meaningful content or "secret" fantasies, and the pattern of women succumbing to his pursuits left him feeling empty, disappointed and shameful.

Freud's early followers elaborated the concept of phallic narcissism (Reich, 1933) as the fixation at the phallic stage of psychosexual development and the associated inability to progress to object-love. Since then, Davies, Benjamin, Stein, Fonagy and others have incorporated more elaborated object relational and intersubjective perspectives into the Freudian theories of psychosexual development and narcissism. They view developmental failures in intersubjective recognition and affect regulation as burdening the normal developmental task of mastering the excessiveness, or 'alien self' aspects of sexual development. Benjamin (2015), for instance, states: "The inability to tolerate the otherness of the sexual and its inevitably high level of arousal manifests as the fear of 'too-muchness', both in intimate relations and in the transference" (p. 42).

Problems with early attachment, and the related difficulties in self and object development, are thus embedded in the development of psychosexuality and manifest as the fear of being overwhelmed by all forms of intimacy, including the sexual experience. Mr. A had been unable to mentalize his own erotic response to his mother's enigmatic messages because the difficulties in the dyad suppressed independent thoughts and feelings. Another major difficulty in his early development had been the lack of a more engaged paternal presence with whom he may have been able to establish secure boundaries between his internalized sense of self and other. He had been deeply disturbed in learning of his father's long-term affair as it further impaired his ability to turn to his father without risking the insecure attachment to his mother.

> A cohesive sense of personal agency can fail to develop, or be crushed in many ways, in sexual trauma, for example.... But agency can also be twisted, suffocated, and destroyed more insidiously, by the failure of the parents to be able to see and recognize the child as an individual in their own right, apart from the parents' own mental scheme of who the child is or should be.
>
> (Slavin, 2010, p. 13)

Thus, Mr. A's sense of self and others was not well established, leaving him unable to use projection with reintrojection to experience the loss of boundaries during sex that would allow for satisfaction of his attachment and sexual yearnings (Fonagy, 2008). The evacuation of his excessive unregulated desire and fantasies into others left him feeling false and inadequate as a man. He described feeling he was on 'auto-pilot' early in treatment and I came to understand his inability to feel mutuality in relationships left him feeling hollow and lifeless. These difficulties also precluded Mr. A from experiencing me as a separate person and led to his experiencing our relationship as 'contractual' until late in the treatment. Through processing the rupture of my analytic reverie, I came to see that I had overestimated our level of intimate engagement due to overlapping blind spots in the analytic field and had confused 'getting understanding' with the transformative experience of being understood (Joseph, 1989).

The enigmatic presence of Mr. A's mother had pulled at my own unconscious eroticized omnipotent fantasies. He reported being very close with his mother, but her presence was illusive; he had not described her in a way that brought her to life in our work. I 'filled in' the absence of a more fully formed maternal representation by seeing her as a mother who may have allowed herself vicarious, competitive pleasure in knowing that her son had not been 'happy in love' for many years. Despite Mr. A's continued fusion with his mother at that juncture in the treatment, it seemed that he had not shared with her details of our work, and this may have fueled my identification and competition with her as I assumed a parallel position in listening to the provocative mix of eroticized yearnings and disappointments in love.

In the session prior to the rupture, Mr. A revealed feeling angry with his mother for criticizing his choice of girlfriends and not choosing "someone more like herself". I again 'filled in' this interaction between us, believing it to be his independent recognition of the mother's erotized narcissistic motivations in criticizing his girlfriends. This led me to feel I had been able to "steal him away" from her, and omnipotently undo the damage I perceived in their narcissistic fusion. I came to believe we colluded in keeping these pleasurable but shame-filled undertows as dissociated "blind spots" in the analytic field that likely echoed his mother's enigmatic and unregulated sexuality. Perhaps the evolution of these blind spots between us was a replication of the parents' blind spots during the husband's affair, with the rupture in the next session perhaps mirroring the 'discovery' of the more than 20-year-long affair along with its undertow on the family.

Mr. A's 'dirty talk' was delivered with a seductive tone that conveyed the physical experience along with the literal meaning of his words. His tone 'invaded' my ears and brought with it unwelcome sexual arousal (Sharpe, 1940). The invasion of my privacy dramatically shifted the gradient of intimacy between us and collapsed my capacity to maintain the distinction between psychic reality and external reality. The overwhelming feelings were difficult to bear; yet as I 'became' what he could not mentalize, I was able to recognize the transgressive trauma that had further overwhelmed his ability to process sexual feelings and fantasies. Brown (2011) reviews psychoanalytic theories on how transformation occurs through projective identification:

> On the level of unconscious phantasy, the analyst's identification with the projection ensures that the analysand experiences him or her as having 'become what others [the patient] believe(s) you are.' It is this unconscious recognition on the patient's part that the analyst has become the projection and can tolerate this experience that creates for the analysand a sense of being authentically understood.
>
> (p. 58)

As I came to reflect on my participation in the unconscious fantasies that had been split off from the analytic field, I was able to listen to his material with fuller access to my reverie. I recognized that the excessiveness of his material led me to be less affectively present and to 'fill in' areas of discomfort with my own unconscious experiences. As described by Akhtar (2013), I began to 'refuse to listen' to material that he was using for instinctual discharge and narcissist stabilization without dissociating myself from our evolving analytic process.

I believe my ability to 'become' his overwhelmed, shamed self-projection, and address my own contributions to our unconscious fantasy, allowed him to talk more openly about his problems with time and missing sessions, and ask me if I remembered the end of our last session. His coopting of my words after I recounted my recollection of the session seemed to be a reenactment of a perverse scenario with his mother in which they had to share all their conscious thoughts to maintain the attachment in their fused narcissistic identifications.

> To remain in loving attachment to his abusive parent the child must dissociate his own reality and his own reality testing capacities, and to hold on to the integrity of his own mind he must forego the love he so craves followed by periods of desolation.
>
> (Davies, 2013, p. 6)

Mr. A perpetuated the perverse scenario in the continuing oscillations of remaining fused with his mother (both interpersonally and intrapsychically) with the necessary splitting off of his own separate reality (manifest as compulsive sexual activity), followed by cycles of foregoing his yearnings for love in order to separate and think his own thoughts (the periods of disappointment in love and lifelessness). His recognition of my 'otherness' was brought to the analytic field when he asked me if I remembered the end of our last session, and as I 'succumbed' to his request, he cycled to his disappointment in not obtaining recognition and love. The empty aloneness then ascendant, he attempted to re-establish his omnipotent narcissistic fusion with me by coopting my words from another interchange in the previous session. This presented me with the complementary choices of the perverse scenario, either again succumbing to him, this time with a denial of my own subjectivity/reality to preserve our attachment (perhaps by minimizing my experience of being coopted) or risk the 'loss of his love' by persisting in my own accounting of the session. My memory of the session as I am writing this paper is that I was aware of the 'doer–done to' (Benjamin, 2004) aspects of our interaction as I persisted in bringing to his awareness my 'version' of the session, while also being aware of the 'third position', that no one could know with complete certainty who had said what in the session. Thus, I exposed us both to the 'unknowableness of mother's interior' (Meltzer, 1971), the essential aesthetic conflict of life, that despite how intimate we can become, we can never fully know each other.

Mr. A seemed to be using the analytic field as a 'first possession', working to establish a 'resting area' (Winnicott, 1971) where he could play with his illusions. I felt he was 'using' (Winnicott, 1969) me as an object who could accept and contain his projections by letting him 'under my skin' without completely losing my self-boundary or invading his, as he experienced anonymous women coming "out of the woodwork" or the seductive mother who wanted him to be with "someone like herself".

> The third part of the life of a human being, a part that we cannot ignore, is an intermediate area of experiencing, to which inner reality and external life both contribute. It is an area that is not challenged, because no claim is made on its behalf except that it shall exist as a resting-place for the individual engaged in the perpetual human task of keeping inner and outer reality separate yet interrelated.
>
> (Winnicott, 1971, p. 6)

The narcissistic identification with mother, and deep ambivalence towards father, evolved to a more defined separation between his self and object representations that could be seen in the shift away from the profound dread of the repetitive dreams of car accidents and fights with guns. The dream of having his own family in a spaceship conveyed his emerging ability to use dreams to link the past with libidinal wishes:

> One might think in Bion's (1962) terms of unmetabolized, erotic beta elements and the kind of alpha dream work that must convert these disparate sensations into a more coherent story line of desire, longing, flirtation, romance, sexuality proper, triumph, disappointment, defeat, and survival.
>
> (Davies, 2013, p. 2)

In Mr. A's reflection on his promiscuity when recounting the 'joke' in which he called a girlfriend a 'slut' and referred to himself as the "mother of all indiscretion", I noted that his split-off overstimulated self-representation onto his girlfriend was better mentalized than the earlier evacuation into the older teacher/analyst representation. With his increased tolerance for separation and fewer blind spots in the analytic field, the emerging intimacy between us was evident as I empathically joined with him in seeing him as "the mother of all indiscretion". I noted the projection of shame onto women in his word choice of 'slut', but I experienced this primarily through reverie. This time, the projection did not invade my self-boundary as the earlier projection onto the older woman representation had, and I could now remain affectively available. He was still partially fused with his maternal representation as the omnipotent 'mother', but he allowed us to reflect together on his humiliating his girlfriend by calling her a 'slut' due to his own shameful self-experience, along with the ineffectiveness ('irony') of that interpersonal strategy. He withstood my/his/our open recognition of his 'sluttiness'. This felt as if we had reached a stage of "interpsychic exchange", defined by Bolognini (2016) as "a natural and shareable process in a condition of mutual understanding and interaction between two human beings" (p. 1).

In the last year of treatment, I noted an evolution in Mr. A's fantasies. Fonagy (2008) and others describe the crucial role of bisexual fantasizes for pleasurable mutuality in normal sexual development. Early in treatment, Mr. A described 'bisexual omnipotence' fantasies of feeling that he was a woman in a man's body, and I felt that fantasy underlying his psychic 'hijack' of my body. This enactment allowed Mr. A to feel arousal 'through' me without threatening his narcissistically fused self and other representation. The omnipotent fantasy may have also been a way to psychically keep his mother and father together and fend off envy of his sisters and father's lover. Towards the end of treatment, he talked about "choosing to follow in his mother's footsteps" in his field of study, seeing himself as separate, but still similar, to his mother. He was able to tolerate the 'otherness' of his mother, and 'bear the guilt of parricide' as he saw himself leaving his parents behind (Loewald, 1979). He had come to mourn the absence of his father's love and give up the melancholic identification with his father as a philanderer, as a 'fallen man' (Butler, 1995). He now recognized he and his father as flawed, but essentially, good men.

These areas of growth in the last year of treatment were reflected in our relationship as an increase in Mr. A's ability to tolerate separation and contain his psychosexual feelings. He shared much less with me about his sexual activity as he seemed increasingly able to 'use' me as an object that he could place outside of his separating subjectivity. We both saw his increasingly differentiated sense of self in his dreams, which he could now use as sources of meaning that linked the past with a wished-for future. With his self and object representations no longer fused as a woman in a man's body, it seemed Mr. A had 'found meaning in the space created by the tolerable absence of the object' (Civitarese & Ferro, 2015). My dream for him was that he would share those pleasurable bisexual fantasies again with a girl like the one he dreamt of in the floating spaceship, settled in a garden reborn from the scorched earth around his home.

Conclusion

Insufficient intersubjective experiences of intimacy early in life can lead to difficulties in tolerating separation and the inherent otherness of sexuality. Without adequate containment, sexual feelings can be experienced as threatening to an insecure attachment and become 'too much' to bear. The fantasies and interpersonal relationships that facilitate mentalization of sexual bodily experiences in normal sexual development can only be employed to the extent that sexual feelings can be experienced without being split off and dissociated.

The analyst's acceptance and processing of split off and projected 'too muchness' can open the possibility of empathic connection and recognition. Through varied use of privacy and intimacy, this empathic connection and recognition can lead to mentalization of relational trauma, sexual transgressions and overwhelming shame. The intimate experience of being recognized as a unique individual whose intolerable experiences are accepted and understood by the analyst can then support the development of self-agency and empathy.

Increasing intimacy in the analytic relationship also brings increasing recognition of the limits of empathy. No gradient of intimacy or mutual recognition can overcome the 'unknowableness' of the maternal body. The acceptance of this existential paradox is also mediated through the varied experiences of privacy and intimacy as they provide further stepping stones in life's journey to achieve intimacy while remaining separate.

Chapter 8

Technology, intimacy and the simulation of intimacy

Todd Essig, Danielle Magaldi and Leora Trub

Numerous technologies afford social relations at a distance. Depending on your point of view, these tools have either severed or liberated intimacy from physical co-presence in contexts as different as family life, friendships, sexual relations, romance and dating, psychotherapy and psychoanalysis, pedagogy and even child- and elder-care. Evolutionary imperatives for attachment, sexual gratification and companionship mediated by cultural practices and neurobiological endowments organized to meet those needs no longer require being bodies together. From texting to FaceTime, with virtual reality (VR) platforms on the horizon, it is no exaggeration to say technologically mediated simulations of traditional physically co-present relationships, i.e. screen relations, are everywhere.

Screen relations specifically reference interpersonal fields where the functional interdependence of individual unconscious and conscious processes are partially determined by the affordances of the technologies being used (Brahnam, 2017; de Wit, de Vries, van der Kamp, & Withagen, 2017; Gibson, 1979).[1] But to what effect? Because we know the functional consequences of screen relations are not the same as physical co-presence even when experiences feel similar (Chavooshi, Mohammadkhani, & Dolatshahee, 2017; Essig, 2015a; Russell, 2015), it is important to ask what is gained and what is lost in screen relations, i.e. what are the consequences of technology mediating intimate experience? This chapter will take up that question. To accomplish the task, following a brief introductory comment about the intended meaning of the term 'intimacy', we will consider the past, present and possible futures of intimacy as experienced through screen relations.

'Intimacy' is a polysemous term requiring specification. It commonly refers both to a quality of a relationship and to one's private interior spaces, both psychological and physical (Rothe, 2018). It can mean both "really, really mine" and "really, really ours". We intend both meanings. Though part of different domains of inquiry, both inevitably imply the other. In fact, contemporary psychoanalysis emphasizes how interpersonal patterning and private experience are isomorphic transformations of each other (Levenson, 1996). Therefore, an inclusive meaning will be most useful for considering what is gained and lost when technologies mediate shared intimate experience.

More specifically, in a recent plenary address to the International Psychoanalytical Association (IPA) annual congress, Levy (2017) described a "true intimate experience" as being when there "are two separate subjects with their sense of otherness preserved, each being themselves, but sharing an emotional experience present in the analytic field" (p. 98). For Levy the pinnacle of intimacy means openly sharing the full range of human emotion, including the unbearable, in one's relationship to self or other rather than having those experiences "evacuated from the mind through action, defensive projective identification, or hallucinations". So, for Levy, moments of intimacy exist on a continuum with 'autistic isolation' on one end and 'narcissistic fusion' on the other. He illustrates the continuum like this: autistic isolation < – > intimacy < – > narcissistic fusion.

Our approach builds on Levy's formulation by making two related changes. First, rather than limiting intimacy to the center of the continuum, we re-describe the center as mutuality and emotional attunement, those times when there is "a shared experience of openness and response" (Levenson, 1974). This midpoint is what Ehrenberg (1992) has called "the intimate edge": "That point of maximum and acknowledged contact at any given moment in a relationship without fusion, without violation of the separateness and integrity of each participant" (1992, p. 424). Second, we adopt a more inclusive and dynamic understanding of intimacy in which it refers to a relationship's capacity for movement across the entire continuum. An intimate relationship is thus one that contains a wide range of emotional experiences and needs, including the asymmetrical and defensive. The more supple the movement across the entire continuum, the more intimate. As illustration, consider an analogy to music. Music can encompass silence and atonality along with melodies and harmonies. Similarly, the range and depth of experience necessary for a relationship to be considered intimate should also include possibilities on both ends of the continuum. Intimacy is more than relationship melodies and harmonies. So, the more fluidly two or more people can move across this continuum, the more intimate the relationship. Exemplars of intimate experience can therefore include when a mother tends to an infant lost in autistic isolation, when lovers omnipotently share moments of narcissistic fusion, and when analytic dyads share regressive or angrily hostile experiences (Pizer, 2014).

In what follows we will be describing changes to intimacy occasioned by the culture-wide acceptance of screen relations as a method for communicating and connecting with each other. When surveying the past, present and future of screen relations, we will be asking whether new technologically mediated intimacies are gains or losses. By exploring intimacy being gained and intimacy being lost, we hope to contribute both to the psychoanalytic understanding of emerging techno-culture and to the larger project of helping construct an inevitably technological future for intimate relationships.

Past: a very brief history of screen relations

The history of when screen relations first entered human experience reveals what happens when a mediating technology gets introduced into an interpersonal field. It shows that there is a significant capacity to experience the presence of other people based on even minimal information, as long as the information is reliable and mimics the interactive temporality of physically co-present exchanges. Such information results in 'telepresence', an illusion of non-mediation in which the experience of being with someone feels as though it were immediate and not mediated by some sort of technology (Lombard & Jones, 2013). And history shows telepresence is driven more by a powerful human need to connect than by technology's marvels, even today's whiz-bang techno-miracles. In fact, as was gauzily sung in old AT&T long-distance commercials, it is not that hard to use interactive technology to *reach out and touch someone.*

The starting date for culture-wide acceptance of screen relations can be set on May 24, 1844, although there were several earlier decades of experimentation and competition among competing approaches. But on that day Samuel Morse, surrounded by government dignitaries at the U.S. Supreme Court building, sat in front of a new-fangled electronic telegraph about to send a message over the first wired link from the capitol. He tapped out the prophetic phrase "what hath God wrought". Almost immediately, just like in a traditional conversation, his interlocutor in Baltimore, MD, replied with the same message. And with this early example of conversational mirroring, the 19th-century fascination with what has been called the "Victorian Internet" took off (Standage, 1998). For the first time in human history, people could instantaneously communicate across distance.

Information started to flow freely. Instrumental applications in commerce and politics rapidly accelerated, helping to transform America into a nation of "manifest destiny" (Howe, 2007). But commerce and politics was not all. Relationships were also conducted over the 'wire'. Marriage ceremonies full of hope and joy, as well as contractual obligations, took place on the wire. By 1879 intimate experiences previously possible only with physical co-presence, but which now took place via technologically mediated simulations of conversation, had entered the public imagination with sufficient force to allow the publication of *Wired Love* by Ella Cheever Thayer (1879). This novel told the story of Nattie and Clem, two telegraph operators who fell in love by sharing dots and dashes without ever meeting in person. And when they did meet after several melodramatic turns, Nattie initially said, "I had more of your company on the wire". The era of simulated intimacy was underway.

The telegraph, unlike letters, was able to temporally mimic what took place when people were bodies together. Operators who experienced that interactive patterning came to feel the presence of others even though they were at a distance, not unlike what takes place today via Skype or FaceTime. Even just interactively sending Morse code back and forth afforded an experience of telepresence, a feeling of being with someone when actually being by oneself. The start of Chapter 2 of *Wired Love* is a wonderful example: "Miss Nattie Rogers, telegraph operator, lived, as it were, in two worlds. The one her office, dingy and curtailed as to proportions, but from whence she could wander away through the medium of that slender telegraph wire, on a sort of electric wings, to distant cities and towns". Nattie teaches us that very little information is required to generate an experience of telepresence so long as it is properly patterned. In addition, and obviously, technological mediation via the telegraph also shows how telepresence limits the richness of experience, implicates different relational processes than the ones used in person, and eliminates the risks and consequences of being bodies together. And what was true for yesterday's telegraph is true for today's texting, audio, video and even virtual reality platforms. Although not as clear with the apparent magic of today's devices, technological mediation always limits the range of intimate possibility while allowing for intimate experience within those limits, intimacies that would otherwise not be possible.

Present: screen relations today (almost)

The technological reconfiguration of intimacy that began with the telegraph is accelerating, many say exponentially (Kurzweil, 2001): it took 50 years for the telephone to reach 50 million users; 22 years for TV; 12 years for cell phones; and two years for Twitter. The geolocation game Pokémon Go reached 50 million users in only 19 days. One problematic consequence of the exponentially accelerating pace of technological development and adoption is that technologies are being deployed much faster than research can possibly happen. As a result, the available research is necessarily limited to statements about what people used to do in the very recent past, not what they do now, resulting in research-based stories about technology use that are frequently lacking in nuance (Essig, 2013; Neri, 2018). Therefore, saying anything useful requires both an as-near-to-the-present-as-possible description of what people are doing, and a willingness to generalize based on experiences present from the very beginning of the technological revolution.

With that caveat in mind, we know that today's screen relations are both compelling and duplicitous. They answer the insistently human call to connect while simultaneously heeding the opposite urge to protect oneself through isolation or merger. On the side of gain, they can afford many of the pleasures and comforts of constant and instantaneous connection. For example, people allowed to text intimates during surgery with local anesthesia end up using significantly fewer opiates for pain relief than both those without access to their phones and those who could distract themselves with a video game (Guillory, Hancock, Woodruff, & Keilman, 2015). But there is loss. Screen relations work their relational magic without the usual consequences and risks. Less is at stake. They allow the experience of being alone together, as Turkle (2011, 2015) has noted. In addition, as is frequently seen in clinical practice, screen relations often leave people feeling vaguely unsatisfied so that when screens go dark there remains an ungratified desire for more. It is no surprise then that screen relations breed screen relations, a fact routinely exploited by social media and technology companies (Alter, 2017) and noted in sensationalized media reports (e.g. Twenge, 2017a). At the extreme, the constant availability of interactive experiences that leave people wanting more, and then more, leads to problematic over-use that sufferers describe as an 'addiction', conveying how their screen relations leave them with the compulsive/impulsive, self-destructive and isolative suffering of a drug addict (Essig, 2012b)

Family and friendships

Even with friends and families, navigating needs for closeness and intimacy includes the challenges of being able to tolerate loneliness, find autonomy and share complicated feelings. Devices offer tempting alternatives. They afford experiences of feeling connected to friends and family without necessarily having to face the more complicated feelings that arise in close relationships. These technologically mediated connections attenuate intimacy by making isolation look like mutuality and attunement. Turkle (2004) noted, "If one is afraid of intimacy yet afraid of being alone, a computer offers an apparent solution: the illusion of companionship without the demands of friendship. In the mirror of the machine, one can be a loner yet never be alone" (p. 21).

The impact of technology on families is enormous but complex, both removing and creating relational obstacles. The constant and instantaneous nature of contact through smartphones provides for the pleasures of abiding connection while blurring boundaries between people, leaving less room for independence. A majority of adults and children check their phones repetitively, feeling an imperative to respond immediately to texts and direct messages (Common Sense Media, 2016). Friends and romantic partners 'chat' back and forth throughout the day (Ohadi, Brown, Trub, & Rosenthal, 2017; Pettigrew, 2009), often coming home at the end of the day to partners or friends they never truly separated from. With casual "how was your day" conversations no longer necessary, people turn to their screens to lessen the resulting conversational discomfort.

For young adults undergoing the transition to college, increased contact with parents and friends can be useful (Ranney & Troop-Gordon, 2012). While gratifying in the short-term, however, being in constant contact does not necessarily translate to feeling close and connected, and in fact may do the opposite (Turkle, 2015; Twenge, 2017b). For example, while the frequency of contact between college students and their parents is on the rise (Hofer & Moore, 2010), the reliance on text-based modes of communication does little to alleviate feelings of loneliness or promote better adjustment during this often difficult transition (Gentzler, Oberhauser, Westerman, & Nadorff, 2011). Meanwhile, the diffusion of boundaries challenges the right to privacy and solitude (Geser, 2006), leaving little room for individuals to cultivate themselves without the input of others who are constantly commenting, 'liking' and influencing the development of one's thoughts, feelings and very identity.

Along with relational boundaries becoming more diffuse and increases in the frequency of connection, barriers to communication and intimacy are rising. Intimacy during family dinners has declined as spaces that used to be reserved for conversation have been replaced by texting under the table while maintaining the illusion of togetherness above it (Turkle, 2015). During meals, school pickup, sporting events and playing in the park, children regard the phone as competing for their parents' attention. Despite feeling badly about it, parents readily admit to checking email instead of talking to their kids during bath time, playtime and dinnertime (Turkle, 2015). A national survey conducted by *Highlights*, a popular children's magazine, found that 'cell phones' was the top response when children were asked what distracts their parents. When asked what would happen if her parents lost their phone, one 9-year-old responded: "They would pay more attention to me" (Joyce, 2014).

Although the mere presence of technological devices does not cause adverse or neglectful parenting (Plowman, McPake, & Stephen, 2010), using technology inevitably divides a parent's attention and leaves less psychic space for interacting with the child. While the phone may theoretically offer a compelling and easy way to maintain contact with other adults when engaged with child care, it simply isn't possible to fully be with one's child and one's friends or co-workers at the same time. Human attention is limited. Caregivers who are highly absorbed with their phones respond more harshly to children's misbehavior (Radesky et al., 2014). Moreover, parental preoccupation with technology has been implicated in higher levels of their children's misbehavior (McDaniel & Redesky, 2018). Such misbehavior may arise from a

> longing for . . . the pleasure of full attention, coveted and rare. These teenagers grew up with parents who talked on their cell phones and scrolled through messages as they walked to the playground. Parents texted with one hand and pushed swings with the other. . . . Previously, children had to deal with parents being off with work, friends, or each other. Today, children contend with parents who are physically close, tantalizingly so, but mentally elsewhere.
> (Turkle, 2011, p. 266)

As we have transitioned into a mode of functioning where being busy and connected is equated with being alive and mattering, we exist in a state of "continuous partial attention", attending as much as possible to as many people or things as possible at the same time. Growing up in this environment, children may follow their parent's lead in learning to stay only partially attentive in order to avoid disappointment (Stone, 2009). In terms of intimacy, parents' continuous partial attention inclines them towards either autistic isolation or narcissistic entitlement while the child yearns for mutuality and attunement. In this way device attachments attenuate intimacy by making it impossible to smoothly flow into mutuality and attunement. Plus, the device then provides solace for disappointments that would not be present if not for the device.

As a result, the very children who have felt snubbed or slighted by their parents' inability to put down the phone cannot themselves put it down. Half of teens openly describe themselves as being addicted to their devices (Common Sense Media, 2016). Young adults increasingly rely on texting to express thoughts and feelings rather than expressing them in person or on the phone (Trub & Barbot, in press), resulting in important communications happening absent nonverbal cues and physical consequence that are necessary for the building of empathy and intimacy (Turkle, 2011). In one study, 67% of people reported checking their phone even without it vibrating and 44% reported sleeping with it on or near their bed so they don't miss an incoming message or call (Smith, 2012). The intensity of our connection to our phones allows for the avoidance of unpleasant internal or external circumstances, as consuming oneself in a device can keep anxiety, sadness or loneliness out of awareness (Cullen, 2011; Trub & Starks, 2017). Denial can also prevail over awareness of how phones may be impacting the potential for intimacy. For example, in one study, even though both teens (41%) and their parents (77%) described feeling that the other is distracted by devices and unable to pay attention when they are spending time together, more than 85% of these same parents and teens indicated that the use of devices has "made no difference in or has even helped their relationship" (Common Sense Media, 2016). Technology really can be quite the trickster.

For some, the new status quo that allows technology to keep people connected but less intimate has reached beyond an acceptable threshold. In his book *Revenge of the Analog*, Sax (2016) argues that there is a revival afoot to return to distinctly human ways of creating and relating to one another, as we are coming to recognize the limitations of our devices. Fighting against the powerful temptation to check the phone for messages when out with friends and loved ones, young adults have devised all kinds of methods for enforcing restraint, for example the "phone stacking game" where a group of friends at a restaurant places their phones in the middle of the table at the start of dinner and whoever looks at their phone before the end of the meal has to pick up the tab (Tell, 2013). Young people today are finding ways to push back against the draw of the phone and expectations of immediate responsiveness, and they are recognizing that in order to shift behavior, external controls may be needed. Intimacy among friends and family may need some help in order to triumph over the seductive allure of easy connection.

Romance and sexuality

Romantic and sexual relationships now exist not only in our bedrooms, but also in our pockets. Smartphones are integral to how we relate and feel close to each other, the way we communicate sexual interest and desire, and how we have sex. Desire and intimacy can no longer be understood apart from the technology we use to experience and express it; mediating technologies are as important to the sexual script as the sexual acts that may or may not follow. Sexual invitations occur via apps, emotional disclosures take place on Snapchat, Instagram and Facebook, and, should we want some safe sexual experimentation from afar, we can sext an interested partner on our lunch break. Whether we march with dispatch into our sexual future or are warily pushed along, technology is now the warp to our erotic weft, part of the very fabric of intimacy.

Although sexual desire seems so fundamental a human need as to be impervious to technology's impact, technology has, in fact, changed how we negotiate sexual desire and intimacy (Smith & Anderson, 2016). We now have instant access to breathtaking amounts of sexual information online, where digital pornography allows us to search for just about any sexual proclivity or curiosity and find a plethora of videos, images, chat rooms or websites devoted to those interests. Instant gratification of desires we may never have even known we had is all right there at our fingertips. And if that doesn't feel real enough, we can don virtual reality headsets to have a multisensory interactive sexual experience without another person. Sexual gratification and experimentation can occur anytime at all. On the hookup scene, mobile dating apps have exploded the sample size of potential sexual partners based on geolocation, promoting a philosophy of "loving the one you're near" in a free market economy of sex and dating (Quiroz, 2013). Traditional sexual intimacies grapple with relationships that begin based on one's coordinates or happen exclusively over a screen.

It's hard to estimate the effects on intimacy when mobile dating is described as "like ordering Seamless" (Sales, 2015). Easy access to heaps of potential partners through apps, the proliferation of digital pornography to suit any fancy, and virtual reality and sexual simulation experiences have changed sex and coupling. Hitting on someone no longer entails overcoming some social and performance anxiety to begin an in-person conversation; instead you "slide into a DM",[2] so that instead of "going back to my place" anyone interested can take conversations from a public online space to direct messaging for a more private and personal touch. On college campuses, the once standard 'booty call', which meant that someone had to call another at home to see if they wanted to meet up to have sex, has been replaced by texting and direct messaging, where partners are readily accessible by smartphones (Goluboff, 2015). One possible benefit to these changes for heterosexual pairings is that women now feel they have greater options for how to establish contact with someone safely if they want to have casual sex (Goluboff, 2015). However, these digital 'conversations' still follow heteronormative gender scripts where men initiate the sexual advance by swiping instead of sweeping a woman off her feet, all in search of the next 'Tinderella' (Hjorth & Lim, 2012; Casado & Lasen, 2014). So while the phone has upset how sexual encounters and intimate contact is initiated, many traditional gender-role norms remain undisturbed within new techno-enabled sexual scrimmages.

While some worry that intimacy is attenuated by technology's new accessibility for sex and instant coupling – why bother dealing with relational challenges when so many other options are a swipe or a click away? – others believe dating apps allow for "networked intimacy" (Hobbs, Owen, & Gerber, 2017). "We have mutual friends, so add me" is the trademark of this networked intimacy propagation, connecting friends of friends over assorted social media apps and forming a type of intimate supernet, increasing social capital and developing loose ties with large numbers of people. Those ties may offer a strong sense of community, security and connection, conjuring intimate feelings and helping us feel a sense of belonging – all of which are important to wellbeing. Intimacy, however, derives from the broader range of experience attendant on face-to-face authentic self-disclosures and affective experiences within the unscripted vulnerability of our social interactions. Social media may offer a strong component of, or a convincing substitute to, intimacy, within the sheer volume of interactions and self-disclosures exchanged, but without the depth and quality of closeness that emerges from mutual, un-manicured, authentic self-expression (Demir, 2015). We may feel connected but still feel lonely or longing.

Romantic partners are using texting, sexting and 'liking' for connecting to each other, and some judge relational intimacy through technology's lens. An attentive, responsive, attuned partner may be one who responds quickly to texts or who consistently 'likes' our Instagram posts. Providing a status update for others to see is now an important way to emotionally disclose and is considered a key component of intimacy (Manago, Taylor, & Greenfield, 2012). And in a couple where going days without seeing or talking with each other may not be unusual, one may feel rejected or abandoned if their partner does not keep up a daily Snapchat streak. As tantalizing as it may be to remove separation and dilute boundaries in sexual and romantic relationships, doing so may jeopardize the intimacy experience. While feeling close from afar has never been easier, feeling close when near has become more difficult.

Coming of age and sexual awakenings

iGen is the first generation to come of age in the smartphone era (Twenge, 2017b). Unlike older generations who integrated technology into previously constructed intimate lives replete with analog procedures for relationships, closeness and sexual desire, iGen is learning intimacy on screen (Magaldi, Appel, & Berler, in press). Their gaming consoles connect them to players who are friends, their hookups occur using the phone, and their friend networks span various social media platforms. They routinely blur differences between physically co-present relationships and those that exist online (Mihailidis, 2014). Such reliance can even morph into dependence. Sometimes the phone itself becomes a love object (Ahuvia, 2005; Trub & Barbot, 2016). It is not surprising that teens describe being without a phone like "standing in public with your vocal cord[s] removed" (Goluboff, 2015).

They experience swirling adolescent change in full online view of each other, such as 'coming out' to friends online before 'irl' (in real life) or tagging someone as 'all glowed up' in response to images of successful 'adulting'. While so called "life on the screen" has always afforded teens the options of trying on various selves (Turkle, 1995), for iGen it is ubiquitous and socially mandatory, affording teens the space to explore different facets of self and form personality structures with near constant feedback from friends. But there are downsides because today's teens still have the same sensitivities to how they are being perceived.

Social comparisons, both upward and downward, are critical for adolescent identity development (Krayer et al., 2008), and social media affords insistent and seemingly unending opportunities for comparison. No surprise that teens who are significant social media users are more likely to believe that others are happier and have better lives (Chou & Edge, 2012; Lup, Trub, & Rosenthal, 2015). Comparisons that might take place in a classroom of 30 students only a decade ago now occur over social media against hundreds, even thousands, of images, posts and curated profiles. It is the fundamental attribution error run amok. Teens see others' social media posts as true representative portrayals rather than skewed highlight reels. When teens compared themselves negatively to others while browsing, the depressive effects can last even after leaving social media browsing, suggesting enduring difficulties regulating mood during and after social media use (Frison & Eggermont, 2016). However, caution is needed. While technology complicates teenage mood regulation and development of self-concept, adolescence naturally marks a time where there is identity confusion and a departure from more positive self-perceptions and an increase in negative self-appraisal (Harter, 2015; Magaldi-Dopman & Park-Taylor, 2010).

Ubiquitous on-screen performance can also pressure some into developing a false self – fabricating or exaggerating those facets of self reinforced by praise from viewers – leading to identity confusion and isolation with significant loss of intimate possibility. While social media promises the benefits of group participation, too often it delivers "feedback overload" (Roback, 2000), scapegoating, targeting and engulfment, which intensify emotional experiences for teens and may increase their sense of alienation and isolation. For those teens experiencing social anxiety and a significant need for social assurance, the risks can be greater, leading to significant problems (Lee-won, Herzog, & Park, 2015).

A false self nurtured online can make friendships and romances precarious. Instead of mutuality and attunement there is often an isolation that comes from feeling inauthentic or, at other times, an engulfment or narcissistic fusion from being whatever others want or expects one to be. The supple movement across different relational configurations that intimacy requires is blocked.

Using the phone to be tethered constantly to others, the confusing boundaries between the curated online self and the real self, and the attachment to the phone itself creates intense emotional conditions during an already acutely volatile time in development. Emotional attunement under these conditions and without the social, facial and vocal contextual cues present 'in real life' is difficult, if not impossible. While teens may socialize and connect to others through social media in a healthy way, they face the possibility of intrusive spikes of anxiety when they are not in contact through social media, depressed mood when comparing oneself with others, and confusion and a loss of self-possession by the narrow range of intimate experience that technology affords.

Clinical intimacies during psychoanalytic treatments

Screen relations, mediated by either audio or video, make treatments and sessions possible that would otherwise not be possible while simultaneously and unavoidably introducing limits on the range of possible intimacies (Russell, 2015; Turkle, Essig, & Russell, 2017). Though sometimes personally difficult, geographically impossible or otherwise impractical to arrange, physical co-presence affords an intimate therapeutic presence (Geller & Greenberg, 2012) impossible to achieve via telepresence. The question for any one case, and for the field in general, is whether the practical gains balance out the lost intimacies. Obviously, that question cannot be reasonably asked without discussing how intimacies are lost when psychoanalytic processes are technologically mediated.

For many years, beginning with the telephone (Saul, 1951; Zalusky, 1998; Aronson, 2000) and continuing with the increasingly wide use of video-conference devices (Carlino, 2011; Lemma, 2017; Scharff, 2013, 2015), technologically mediated simulations of in-person relating have been used to provide psychoanalytic care when someone is ill, traveling for business, on vacation or unable to find a local therapist, as well as used as a way to expand one's practice worldwide. It has been a "better than nothing" solution in those situations when a patient, or analyst, relocates and the dyad wants to maintain continuity. However, this practice is becoming increasingly routinized so that screen relations have moved from a "better than nothing" creative solution for difficult clinical situations to a new normal in which screen relations are treated as good-enough everyday practice. Some even consider screen relations based treatments to be functionally equivalent replacements, such as when used for purposes of a training analysis (Essig, 2015b; Essig & Russell, 2017). This widespread adoption is taking place despite relatively little attention to how screen relations influence and attenuate the range of technologically mediated intimacies.

The available research avoids direct attention to the intimacies lost due to process limitations inherent in available technological affordances. Instead, a rationale for routine screen relations based treatments has been developed based on illustrations of psychoanalytic process during recordings, transcripts or process notes (Scharff, 2013, 2015). What took place is searched for evidence of a psychoanalytic process. When such process is found, screen relations based treatments are declared good enough. Sometimes in-person and on-screen session transcripts are compared to see if people can see the difference. Again, when no difference is found claims of good-enoughness are made (de Setton, 2015). But scant attention is paid to limits, to what might have occurred but could not.[3]

Furthermore, demonstrations of technologically mediated psychoanalytic process should neither surprise nor be given more weight than they deserve, and certainly not be used to deflect attention away from understanding lost intimacies. The fact is that the fundamental human need to connect with others has always made it easy for technology to capture the heart, even with primitive technologies like when Nattie and Clem, our fictional telegraph operators, fell in love over the wire. As a result, it is no longer clinically useful to show that technology can carry some clinical intimacy. It would be surprising, shocking even, if there were no such demonstrations of mediated psychoanalytic process. The important questions are elsewhere, in understanding clinically significant experiences and interactions technological mediation cannot afford. For example, as Russell (2015) wrote, "Loving, as well as destructive, fantasies . . . have no potential to be enacted" (p. 39). Going on to quote a patient, "When you share a physical space, even if you don't act it out, there is always the potential to touch, whether that means kicking or kissing" (p. 39). These differences in what the contexts afford are important. What cannot happen, or happen in the same way, is of significance.

There is another frequently invoked rationale for routine screen relations: first-person accounts from participants attesting to the value, credibility or intensity of the experience. Because the intimacy feels so powerful, some say the treatment is good-enough. Of course, participant experiences are important. However, those experiences are loosely connected to the actual functional consequences of screen relations based treatments. Plus, the technology is actually designed to make the simulations feel the same even though the consequences are radically different, like what happens in a sophisticated flight simulator. Using first-person accounts are particularly problematic guides to clinical decision-making because intimacies on screen sever the usual connection between eventual consequence and the feeling of the moment. Representations with a digital provenance tend to be replaceable cross-sections of the current moment lacking a narrative structure meaningfully extending across time (Hartman, 2017). For example, Russell (2015) noted that many participants find screen relations based sessions less memorable with clinicians relying on note-taking more so than with in-person treatments. Feelings, even when same or similar, don't have the same consequences in the different contexts. Another example is a randomized controlled trial (RCT) comparing video-delivered and in-person intensive short-term dynamic psychotherapy for the treatment of medically undiagnosed pain (Chavooshi et al., 2017). Both groups reported the treatments to be equally credible and satisfying. However, the in-person group had significantly less pain. In addition, the in-person group showed "significant decreases in depression, anxiety and stress as well as a greater increase in emotion regulation functioning, mindfulness and quality of life" (p. 133). The functional consequences of the two treatments were fundamentally quite different even with similar reports of participant experience.

Lost intimacies can be found by looking at how various psychoanalytic processes are altered or blocked in screen relations. We will look at three, but others can easily be found just by looking. Consider first Winnicott's classic observation that a psychoanalyst's role includes providing a "facilitating environment" in which maturation and healing can take place. This does not happen in the same way in screen relations based treatments. Remote patients must in large measure provide their own facilitating environment rather than having it be provided by the therapist (Russell, 2015). They perch on their chair or couch, not ours. Sometimes it's their bed or car, or a random hotel. It's their tissue when a tear appears. They click to open an image, a rather different experience than coming to and leaving a caring other's special space, one that holds and facilitates growth. While this might not attenuate moments of intimacy when the relationship is in a period of mutuality and attunement, i.e. when it is at the center in our continuum of intimacy, possibilities are truncated and intimacies lost when the going gets tough. During those regressive moments of isolation or fusion, patients benefit from being held by an environment provided by the analyst yet created by the patient – something routine technological mediation does not afford.

For example, a patient in the depths of negative transference spent several sessions seething in a mostly silent tantrum. As the sessions ended she grabbed a large handful of tissues from the box on the side-table. She then clutched them tightly walking to the subway before shoving them into her purse. Later she recounted that holding the tissues helped remind her that her hostility would not kill her analyst, that she really didn't want him dead, that both would survive her rage. The clump of tissues squeezed in her hand reminded her that her murderous fantasies were inside, not part of external reality. Self and other were different. The facilitating environment had done its job. Because of this, rage and defensive isolation had become part of the intimacy two separate people shared in this treatment. But had there not been a shared external reality the necessary differentiation would likely not have taken place for two reasons. First, there would have been no shared outer reality to contrast with and illuminate the presence of inner reality. Second, the regressive rage would have been too terrifying to experience in the first place. Technological mediation does not afford the possibility for a full range of intimacy in part because screen relations often include a joint effort, a collusion of sorts, to incline treatment towards the attuned and mutual (Essig, 2013). Dyads truncate experience to keep the relationship viable because remote treatments not inclined towards the center of the intimacy continuum often leave participants alone in the absence of the other. They sit alone with a technology that can no longer afford the experience of telepresence because both participants are no longer working to construct that experience.

Another place to find lost clinical intimacies is differences in how attention is mobilized in screen relations in comparison to being bodies together. These differences in attention result in clinically consequential differences in analytic listening and possibilities for reverie. Screen relations require focused attention on the device, be it screen, speaker or headphones, and compel continuous partial attention while inevitably presenting confusing mediation artifacts. That we can feel the presence of a technologically mediated other requires attentional work unnecessary with physical co-presence where one encounters an interpersonal field so rich one can only avoid it with tremendous effort.

More specifically, experiencing the presence of a remote other requires filtering out relationally extraneous distractions present in the separate environments. One analyst told Russell (2015) during her ethnographic interviews with remote treatment participants that "one of the ways I had to adjust was to not be curious about that [the patient's different space] so that I could just concentrate on what she was telling me" (p. 18). Plus, the devices themselves compel attention, which also must be managed. Even when email, texting and social media programs are closed, they are lurking there in the same machine creating an interpersonal shadow that must be attentionally avoided. Another therapist Russell interviewed said, "I found myself wondering all the time what my email was. I think the nature of the device encourages us to think about multi-tasking". Another confessed, "I'm ashamed to admit to surreptitiously checking my email during a session" (Russell, 2015, p. 131). Also, dropped connections and distortions like time-delays and pixelization are common. Russell recounts one particularly poignant example of a dropped connection in the midst of a patient sharing intense emotions: "The disruption to the flow of our interaction and the distress caused by the abrupt loss of connection felt terribly intense and violent for both of us. It took some minutes to reconnect, and by then the session could not be resumed where we left off. The tear in the fabric of the session was impossible to repair" (2015, p. 128). Furthermore, even when devices work as intended, as Brahnam (2017) clearly articulated, mediation artifacts are "inevitably introduced by the transmission process" that "have the tendency of perturbing and shoving aside the unconscious expressions of human subjects, producing impressions that have nothing to do with the subject yet are often unconsciously confused with him" (p. 139).

Contrast this with open, receptive analytic attention. For example, Ogden (2004) wrote the "analyst's task is to generate conditions that may allow the analysand – with the analyst's participation – to dream the patient's previously undreamable and interrupted dreams. A significant part of the analyst's participation in the patient's dreaming takes the form of the analyst's reverie experience" (p. 857). Intimacies of all sorts grow in such reveries anchored in a shared relational and physical space. But the open receptivity to self and other that reverie requires is necessarily strangled by the attentional demands screen relations require. Unfortunately, and unlike concepts amenable to dialectical paradox (Hoffman, 1998; Stern, 2009), human attention is finite and singular. Attention does not allow both-and solutions. One either adopts a stance of focused attention screen relations require while also struggling against the continuous partial attention technology wants, or maintains the open receptive attention psychoanalytic listening deserves. Consequently, attempts at shared reverie in screen relations would simply leave participants, again, alone in the absence of the other.

A final example of lost intimacies worth noting – and there are many more, all you have to do is look – is in the relationship between implicit processes involving bodily and emotion-based relational knowledge of how to be with someone, and symbolic interpretive processes (Stern et al., 1998). When people are bodies together, procedural and episodic memory line-up or, in other words, states of being encompass states of mind (Russell, 2015). But in screen relations there is a disjunction between what one does to stay engaged via the mediating technology and the telepresence fueled narrative of an empathic, caring relationship enduring across time and distance. An intimate narrative conflicts with the felt, lived experience of being an isolated body.

The following vignette illustrates implicit relational intimacies lost when relationships are conducted on screen. The patient is a pathologically affable, and extremely successful, middle-aged *road warrior* with four children. He travels for business at least three weeks each month. Most sessions are therefore conducted via a mediating technology. During this session he says he feels like he's missing out and doesn't like being a cyber-dad but is stuck with this life. He says he does appreciate being able to say goodnight to his kids via FaceTime but it's not the same. The session is moving along exploring these feelings when he pauses and says, "It's weird to be talking to you with the same screen I use with them . . .

hell, it's also where I work . . . watch movies . . . uhm, even porn . . . all here . . . the same damn screen, if I let myself relax everything blurs together". Something is brewing. The dyad is moving from what the Boston Group (Stern et al., 1998) called a "pregnant phase" to a "weird phase" when he then asks with surprising affective power, "How about you?" The therapist who is also using a multi-function device pauses feeling the affective heat of what's become a "now moment". He responds, "I feel you need me to be like you, struggling to keep you in mind despite all the other ways I use my screen". "Hhmmm," he says, "like with my kids, we pretend . . . but it sucks not being together". The therapist responds by breaking the illusion their relationship requires, "Sometimes, both of us, pretend our relationship is good enough but it's often just better than nothing, at least in treatment we don't need to pretend, we can feel the loss . . . both of us". He responds, "But I need to pretend . . . or I just get too lonely" and he starts to cry. What makes this into a "now moment" of intersubjective meeting was breaking that illusion of telepresence to acknowledge they really weren't together, that he's not really putting his kids to bed when on the road. This now moment makes clear how screen relations include loss and illusion, something both participants feel, yet often collude to ignore. Had this now moment been missed, as frequently happens, it would have reinforced acceptance of the illusion screen relations require. The dyad would have colluded to avoid awareness of loss and limits.

Thus, there are many reasons why it is crucial to be aware of lost intimacies when deciding whether or not to provide treatment remotely. One is that relationships are built from different processes when relating through technology, than when people engage directly with a physically co-present person. These different relational processes stem from the unavoidable fact that technology's promise – you can be anywhere anytime with anyone without loss – is an illusion. As a result, loss and limits are inevitable and we cannot afford to ignore them. Second, being bodies together affords unique risks and outcomes. After all, if you can never be physically dropped, you can never really feel hugged and held, which is a different experience than being constantly quasi-anxious about the connection itself dropping. Third, with physical co-presence one can never specify what might be clinically significant in the comparably more powerful and rich stimulus array of being bodies together. Consequently, being aware of lost intimacies and bringing them into the clinical relationship just may be the best way to provide care at a distance when it becomes necessary to do so. And with such awareness, screen relations based treatments just may be able to remain a better-than-nothing solution for exigent clinical circumstance, as they were always intended to be.

Future: ready or not, here it comes, and it's already here

Now that *Future Shock* (Toffler, 1970) has given way to *Present Shock* (Rushkoff, 2013) where we actually live in the future of exponentially expanding technological options, no question is more important than "how do we make choices today that will result in a world we want to live in?" (O'Reilly, 2017, p. x). No one (we hope) wants to lose intimacy to rampaging technological development in any of the domains surveyed. Yet such an unintended consequence is more than merely possible. Due to artificial intelligence (AI), including emotional and social intelligence, combining with virtual reality (VR) and robotics, the future will be replete with opportunities for artificial intimacy (the other AI), such as fully functional sex-bots and on-screen therapy-bots. In fact, early versions of those two options are already available with the empty promise of everything you want whenever you want it (Essig, 2017). But intimacy's future is not yet written. We still have a say in the central question of whether technologically mediated relating becomes an end in and of itself or facilitates intimacy in non-technological spaces. There is still time to advocate for the analog; recognize the power of good, old-fashioned non-mediated intimacy, and insist on preserving opportunities to have it.

In a dystopian future to be avoided, machines will provide child- and eldercare, at least for the economically privileged. Nannies will become as obsolete as taxi drivers. With more (all?) of life recorded and shared on increasingly sophisticated social media sites the bonding pleasures of shared memories will get lost in an overwhelming digital archive of what 'really' happened. Thanks to advances in VR and teledildonics, people will have interactive sexual experiences connecting only to technology, not other bodies. And with further developments in robotics, sex-bots will make it so that the bodies with which one connects will be made of silicon and programmed to satisfy both physical and emotional desires. Of course, when any of these 'relationships' cause problems all one will have to do is sit down at a screen for a session with a 3-D, photo-realistic therapy-bot who remembers everything you say, is programmed to be optimally 'empathic' and, if you want, looks just like your first-grade teacher who was always unusually kind to you. Irresistible familial, sexual and therapeutic artificial intimacies will become routine. Technology will meet all needs for intimacy. Life will be perfect, at least from the perspective of those selling these amazing gadgets.

But such a future of artificial intimacy, one in which being biological bodies together ceases to have significant relational value, will not come about because of technological advances. After all, the same technologies might be productively used to help the over-worked, comfort the lonely and even help couples increase their intimacy by solving sexual problems with virtual sex partners or educators in a non-threatening way. The difference in the future will be made by us. What we expect from each other relative to what we will cede to machines will tell the tale. Unfortunately dystopian dangers lurk in seemingly innocent trends where people unreflectively relate to and through machines rather than directly with each other.

For example, many families have already found ways to affectionately incorporate Alexa and Siri into their lives, first calling upon them by name to offer a playlist or fill in gaps in the dinnertime conversation and then jokingly – or not – telling a loved one, "Alexa would never talk to me that way!" Children hearing this will grow up expecting devices to mediate relationships between people. They will be primed to develop ever deeper emotional attachments to devices and not to each other, and technologies will be developed to provide those attachments.

In sexuality consider web camming, a multi-billion dollar industry daily engaging thousands of webcam performers and hundreds of thousands of viewers. Innumerable sexual practices are viewed live that include real-time conversation and exchanges with the models. With Bluetooth enabled sex toys and synchronized haptic feedback, models are developing the technological capacity to reach out and touch their viewers, and be touched in return. While the models are just trying to make a living from the users seeking pleasure and company, they are also paving the way to a world where comforting loneliness and gratifying sexual desire will routinely take place via machines.

And in our psychoanalytic corner of the world, therapists routinely providing care on screen are also inadvertently paving the way for acceptance of both artificially intelligent psychotherapy programs, so-called therapy-bots and artificial intimacy in general. We are teaching people that sufficient empathy and intimacy can be found on screen for the most profound of personal transformations we strive to achieve in our work. Routine screen relations based treatments inadvertently communicate the powerful message that being bodies together is just not that important and that profound personal growth can be found on screen. Should that happen it is only a question of time before the technologists will simulate what we do, or at least nearly enough to qualify as routine, good-enough practice, so that 'therapeutic intimacy' will result from person-machine interactions without the presence of a human therapist.

Notes

1 Affordance is a concept from the study of perception relevant to understanding technology use first formulated by J.J. Gibson (1979) who wrote, "The affordances of the environment are what it offers the animal, what it provides or furnishes, either for good or ill" (p. 56). The basic idea is that humans do not perceive the world by taking in disembodied information that is then related to a pre-existing representational structure. Instead, people perceive the world's action potentials. Or, in other terms, we take in the world based on opportunities to fulfill desires and manifest intentions.

2 On social media platforms, DM refers to 'direct message'. It is a private communication between two or more people who had been interacting in public.

3 To see the limitations of this research, consider someone doing psychoanalysis in the food court of a local mall, a clearly absurd but still illustrative example. Let's say transcripts of those "treatments" were studied and evidence found for a psychoanalytic process. Could the claim then be made that "mall analysis" was good-enough?

Chapter 9

Psychoanalytic intimacy

Christie Platt

When Hagai Levy created the television series *In Treatment* in 2005 for Israeli audiences, he had no idea that it would become wildly successful. For nine weeks, audiences were treated to the voyeuristic pleasure of seeing the same four patients, one for each episode, in therapy sessions with their psychologist, Paul Weston. On the fifth day each week, Paul Weston had a quasi-therapy/consultation to discuss these patients with his own supervisor. Because he had his office in his house, audiences were also privy to the difficulties he was having in his personal life. The show was first adapted for American audiences and eventually for countries as diverse as Serbia, Brazil, Russia, Japan and Macedonia. Since its inception, it has been aired in one form or another in over 70 countries around the world. When asked how he came up with the concept, Levy (cited in Gilbert, 2010) said:

> I have been a patient most of my life, going to psychotherapy of various kinds, and I actually studied psychology before I went to film school – my first degree is in therapy. And I always found myself as a director interested more in intimate situations much more than big productions. And I was thinking 'what could be the most intimate thing in the world?' For me that happened to be therapy.
>
> (p. ii)

So, what makes psychotherapy or psychoanalysis so intimate? Is it as intimate for the analyst as it is for the patient given that only the patient reveals the details of their interior world and everyday life? Patient and analyst certainly create a private and confidential world together in order to speak of matters that will enable the patient to lead a freer, more satisfying life. During the course of therapy, the two will discuss not only the aspects of a patient's life that are of obvious significance but also the most trivial events that may somehow enable some unconscious belief to emerge that sheds insight into the inner workings of the patient.

But how to define intimacy? And is it even desirable in a world run rife with boundary violations? Throughout the history of psychoanalysis, the concept of psychoanalytic intimacy has stirred anxious self-reflection and reflexive opposition to its desirability. Whether or not authentic intimacy can truly exist continues to be a question of debate. This chapter seeks to address these questions as well as the multiplicity of ways that psychoanalytic intimacy might manifest itself.

Dictionary interpretations of intimacy

The *New Oxford American Dictionary* provides four possible meanings for the word 'intimacy', the first of which is 'a private cozy atmosphere' as in: 'the room had a peaceful sense of intimacy about it'. Most consulting rooms seek to achieve such an atmosphere. Freud's office, with its carpets, artifacts and even his dogs, created the prototype for the analytic space. His consulting room was adjacent to his apartment and was chockablock full of things he loved; there was no effort to be neutral or abstinent when it came to the office where he spent his days. Office décor is one of the most personal expressions about the analyst that the patient will see yet it is remarkable how little the patient actually does see. It is not uncommon for a patient to say after several years of treatment, "Have you always had that picture?" Something has changed in the patient or the relationship when that picture or object suddenly becomes visible.

The cozy atmosphere of the consulting room may contribute to the patient's ability to achieve the second part of the definition: 'an intimate remark' as in: "Here she was sitting swapping intimacies with a stranger". This is indeed the nature of analysis, with one notable proviso: the analyst does not swap his or her own stories with patients. Only the patient seeks to reveal herself while speaking as freely as possible about her thoughts, feelings and the events of her life. Meanwhile, the details of the analyst's life are (generally) not revealed.

Let us consider the analytic situation more closely. One person enters the consulting room, lies down on a couch and begins to reveal her most delicate feelings, closely held secrets and life stories, many of which have never been uttered before. The analyst, meanwhile, sits directly behind the patient, listening and occasionally commenting or interpreting what is heard. In a sense, free association is akin to meditating out loud, in the presence of a witness. Together, the analytic dyad attempts to take the 'profane' dross of daily life and spin it into the 'sacred' gold of understanding. To do this, the analyst must maintain a sense of separateness, keeping in mind that these meetings are for the benefit of the analysand, who places herself in a vulnerable position, both physically and psychically.

Although it may not seem so to the patient, the analyst also prepares for a demanding emotional encounter whose outcome is unclear. As Poland (2017) writes:

> For as much as I want to do my work, as much as I enjoy doing my work, as much as I believe that the likelihood of success justifies the pains ahead, still there is something else I also know. And that is that whatever else happens, this new analysis is going to go into areas I don't want to enter, into fears

> I would rather keep hidden away. And I know that whatever they will be, they will not be what I could predict or even guess at the start. What will make me wish I were somewhere else will come unexpectedly, from around a corner. (p. 84)

Whatever the outcome of the analysis, both analyst and patient will inevitably be transformed in unforeseeable ways by their relationship.

Returning to the third definition offered by the *Oxford American Dictionary*, intimacy is also defined as a 'closeness of observation or knowledge'. This too resembles the nature of psychoanalysis as both analyst and analysand develop an ever more nuanced and deep understanding of the patient's interior world. While it is evident that the analyst will come to know a great deal about his patient, the patient may know far more about the analyst than is often acknowledged. With the frequency of sessions, the analytic pair really learns to 'live together' throughout the seasons over a period of months or years (Edward Kushner, personal communication, March 17, 1994). There are good days, bad days, insightful days and sterile days. This quotidian intimacy is unique to analysis. Especially today, many people will spend quality time with their analyst that does not exist anywhere else in their lives.

The final definition offered by the dictionary suggests that intimacy is a euphemism for 'an intimate act, especially sexual intercourse'. Here is analytic intimacy run amok in which the conditions that were described above have overwhelmed the capacity of one, or both, of the participants to maintain a therapeutic relationship, in the service of the patient's successful therapeutic outcome. The parameters safeguarding both analyst and patient from the yearnings for closeness that arise in such an atmosphere have never been perfect. Yet, if the conversations between analyst and patient are too formal and restricted, can anything happen in the hour that is alive or authentically meaningful?

As the television show *In Treatment* unfolded, the intimate conversations that took place between Dr. Paul Weston and his patients in the consulting room did, in fact, become far too 'intimate', breaching the parameters that Eissler delineated in 1953 that were intended to create a safe holding environment for both analyst and patient. When Dr. Weston's personal life begins to fall apart in Season One, Paul (as his patients called him) loses his ability to remain committed to helping his patients understand themselves. Instead, he became invested in helping them by becoming a participant in their lives, infusing the sessions with his own unconscious needs and desires. The exquisite empathy that he had for his patients, initially a force for good, became corrupted as he began to use his privileged access to their inner worlds to fulfill his own needs. Such are the dangers that accompany the analyst and patient as they engage in private conversations that seek to provide relief for the patient.

Historical and theoretical perspectives

As psychoanalytic theory has evolved, so has the role of intimacy, although it is rarely discussed as such. Articles about the role of intimacy proliferated in the early 1970s, a time when social and political revolution had penetrated the entire culture in response to the Vietnam War. Timothy Leary captured the American zeitgeist when he coined the phrase, "Question Authority". The humanistic movement emerged as an antidote to the elitist, 'analyst-knows-all' approach that had dominated psychology in the 1950s. Carl Rogers's (1942) 'client-centered therapy' became popular. The therapist was no longer the repository of the answers. Instead, he/she reflected back to the 'client' (who was now called 'client' rather than 'patient') what the patient had just said, in the belief that wisdom could be gleaned by the client herself. Kohut's (1977) empathy for the patient's narcissistic vulnerabilities ushered in an era where previously 'unanalyzable' patients were now thought to be treatable.

In a seminal article, Levenson (1974) re-examined the concept of intimacy. In its earliest literary usage, he posited that intimacy is a private experience that resides within as "the most private and unrevealed parts of the person" (p. 360). During the early 1970s, intimacy was evolving into an interpersonal concept that described the "ambiance of engagement or closeness between therapist and patient which characterizes the 'positive therapeutic alliance' – that state of good intent without which no degree of virtuosity nor depth of experience of the therapist can prevail" (p. 359). Prior to this time, patients and analysts alike shared a myth that both were perfectible. With enough work, neuroses could be resolved and transference and countertransference distortions could also be clarified. The idea of the analyst as a blank screen or tabula rasa began to seem increasingly archaic as well as unattainable. In the post-modern world, it was becoming increasingly evident that the analyst is not, and never was, a completely neutral entity.

The interpersonal, intersubjective and relational models provided alternative ways of viewing therapeutic relationships. As Levenson pointed out, once the idea of the analyst and patient being able to expunge their neuroses and transference/countertransference distortions was debunked, spontaneity and authenticity came forth, with all the consequent potential for messiness but also for growth. One could say that there was an increasing recognition that full knowledge of one's unconscious processes by either party was impossible. Instead, acceptance of the foibles of both parties seemed not only more realistic, but also more therapeutic. "Rather than decontaminating the relationship, the effort becomes to experience it without mystification; to see it as it is, without trying to change or improve it" (p. 363). Levenson was adamant in saying that the analyst "must not use himself as a tool to lever the patient into change" (p. 365). He went even further:

> "All psychodynamic interpretations, just as all metapsychologies, become in the end, acts of countertransference." Patients do not change because they have received new knowledge of themselves by dint of clever interpretations, rather they change with the experience of interpersonal resonance that allows stored information to be repatterned.
>
> (p. 367)

I would add that this resonance takes place in the analyst as well, and to me it constitutes one example of the moments of intimacy that take place in a session.

Shane and Shane (1997) suggest that the boundaries and possibilities for intimacy with a patient depend greatly on the diagnosis of the patient, particularly whether or not the patient sees others as self-objects or as distinctly separate objects. When a person views others as self-objects, they are appreciated for their ability to support and maintain the subject's self and to achieve self-regulation and self-righting. The authors contrast this with intersubjective relatedness, "wherein the other is experienced by the subject as not only psychologically separate and distinct, but also as a person in his or her own right, with his or her own goals and aspirations, and with an inner world the subject longs to share in intersubjective closeness" (p. 74). With patients who use the analyst primarily as a quasi-auxiliary ego and provider of emotional supplies, there is a need to establish firm boundaries. In this situation, the analyst may feel frustrated and angry at being used in such a utilitarian manner. A strong countertransferential temptation to make the patient aware of the analyst as a person in her own right may occur. To feel used merely as a self-object can make the analyst feel belittled and resentful and even sadistic.

On the other hand, patients who exhibit concern and understanding for the analyst may also stimulate a wish in the analyst for a deeper, more mutual relationship. Along the continuum of more interpersonal or relational analyses, the boundaries are more fluid, the guardrails less well-marked. If one is seeking what Guntrip referred to as the "moment of real meeting" (cited in Ehrenberg, 1974, p. 427), a time when the distortions of transference and countertransference have been dissolved and the analyst and analysand can meet face to face as two human beings, what has happened to make that moment possible? Yerushalmi (2013) equates intimacy with moments of meeting and says that these moments occur when "two people establish spontaneous, active, and nonverbal contact, thereby broadening and deepening their relationship and their understanding of it. This is a special opportunity in which an authentic, tangential encounter occurs between them, unintentionally and unexpectedly" (p. 682). But he cautions that these moments may also heighten the desire to be 'emotionally touched and understood' in the therapist as well as the patient, something that is not often discussed among analysts, to their detriment. There are times, with certain patients in particular (Schafer, 1995), when analysts can experience profound loneliness in their work. Often, this can produce unconscious avoidance of the patient, manifested as a dissociative boredom, sleepiness and helplessness. Without mourning what we cannot, and should not, expect to get from our relationship with our patients, we run the risk of all manner of unconscious enactments that may be quite harmful, especially if they never surface to a conscious level that allows for analysis.

When I started my psychoanalytic training in a classical, ego-psychology based institute, we had a seminar in which we were asked whether we thought we would have had the same analysis if we were to have had a different analyst. I thought the idea was absurd, "Of course not!" The personality and responses of the analyst to me would be so specific that even if I had the same conflicts to explore, the way they would have been explored and how I would have felt doing so would have been completely specific as well. I wondered then, as I do now, if that question came from a time when analytic neutrality and abstinence were thought to be possible. When I started my training in the mid-1990s, I was told by a supervisor that I should refrain from making so many interpretations (not that they were really interpretations at that point in my career), possibly only one or two per hour would be ideal. As I read my session notes to another supervisor, she simply said, time after time, "I wouldn't have said that". In my own way, I was trying to figure out how to be an analyst, but also myself. If I couldn't be at least somewhat authentic during the hour, I would also be unable to think, my thinking apparatus paralyzed by "I wouldn't have done that".

But I had also studied in a humanistic psychology program where we were all encouraged to 'share' our ideas and feelings whenever we felt like it. That could devolve into an egalitarian pandemonium of advice. During that time, I sought individual therapy for the first time. It was shortly after my father died and I had received two referrals; both therapists came highly recommended. The first woman I met with had an office in a rundown building in an industrial part of town. The room where we met was painted a sort of sea green that reminded me of administrative offices in a decrepit elementary school. However, she listened for a long time and acknowledged simply that this seemed to be a confusing time for me and I seemed to be somewhat at sea. I left the encounter miserable, but with the feeling that I had been accurately seen. I had a feeling of great relief about that. The meeting had been intimate in that I had felt free to say things that I hadn't expressed to anyone else, things that I didn't even know I felt yet.

The other therapist could have come from central casting with her white hair, deep blue eyes and beautifully embroidered ethnic shawl. She said, "I remember how hard it was for me when my father died". I felt her empathy and her wish to ease my pain, but I also felt that I didn't want to think about her father; I didn't know her, so how could she already imagine that she knew how to relate to me about my father? I needed the spaciousness of the silences, the quiet feeling of my pain being held but not intruded upon, and the interpretations that allowed me to access my unconscious and to discover things about myself that I didn't know before. The work felt free from dogma and from the intrusiveness of an overly involved other.

In 1974, Ehrenberg applied Martin Buber's theory of the 'interhuman' (Buber, 1958) to psychoanalysis. Buber said that this feeling of being human together exists only in the dialogue that two people have together, not in either individual or even in the dyad alone. She cites Winnicott (1960b) as well, whose belief that creating a safe 'holding' environment would allow a patient to reveal his or her 'true self'. She introduced the concept of the 'intimate edge' or "that point of maximum and acknowledged contact at any given moment in a relationship without fusion, without violation of the separateness and integrity of each participant" (Ehrenberg, 1974, p. 425). By staying focused on the quality of attunement between the analytic pair, both members can identify defenses as they arise as well as different levels of engagement in the willingness to connect. The content of the patient's productions and the level of engagement between the analytic pair moves back and forth between figure and ground. In her formulation of the intimate edge, Ehrenberg stresses that "intimacy is something that must be actively created" and that "the mutual focus on the difficulties involved in this collaborative effort becomes the medium of the therapeutic process" (p. 435). Rather than being something to abstain from, psychoanalytic intimacy becomes the healing balm of the therapeutic process. Moreover, this intimacy can contribute to the analyst's growth as well, and if the patient knows that, this knowledge can be a catalyst for even more change in the patient. She does not address the question of whether part of the analyst's motivation for choosing this profession has to do with the opportunity for the analyst's healing.

This opportunity for a mutually created intimate edge can also present a slippery slope towards a sort of therapeutic 'mis-involvement'. Bollas (2006) worried that in the more recent rush towards engagement, analysts have forgotten the importance of listening carefully to patients. He says:

> In recent years I have been concerned by a surprisingly widespread lack of interest on the part of therapists and analysts about what the analysand is actually saying. The crucial early words of a session, the unconscious selection of topics, the patterns of ideas that reveal themselves (eventually) through the movement from one topic to another, the ring of certain phrases, the evocative and ramifying effect of a single word, and the far-reaching suggestion of a metaphor are of so little interest to many clinicians that these features are either not recalled or overlooked.
>
> (p. 714)

Bollas proposes the idea of 'perceptive identification' which is based on the self's ability to perceive the object as a thing-in-itself. If the self can do this, then it can enjoy the object's qualities and be nurtured by the integrity of the object. The more it can perceive the object-in-itself, the more it celebrates the object as different from the self. This model presupposes the *jouissance* of difference (not similarity) and implicitly appreciates the separateness of the object. In this he echoes Winnicott's (1960b) sentiment that it is very important, except when the patient is regressed to earliest infancy and to a state of merger, that the analyst shall not know the answers except in so far as the patient gives the clues.

There is a continuing debate as to whether the analyst must have experienced what her patients' have in order to truly understand them. This often comes up in the field of addictions where people say that you have to have been an alcoholic to treat one. In reality, it is of course impossible to have had every experience in the world, although the analyst uses her experiences every day in the effort to enter the patient's world. When I listen to a patient, I find that pictures begin to form in my mind of the various characters/internal objects that are being described. I visualize houses, summer afternoons, high school teachers and so forth as I try to enter into the patient's world. Invariably, this leads to my own associations to the sounds of birds and the smell of freshly cut grass from my own summer afternoons. As the patient continues, I start to imagine what the person felt like in these circumstances and there is an interplay between the patient's free associations and my own. The efforts I am making are stimulated by the patient's thoughts and memories, but invariably I am revisiting different parts of my life that have often lain dormant for years. Inevitably, the circumstances of the patient's memories veer off from my own and as I follow them in my mind, new insights into my own life emerge as well. Later, as I reflect upon the hour, I will process what the patient said and what I dredged up from my associations. Contemplating both sets of associations is a synthetic process that allows for the re-patterning, described earlier as part of the experience of resonance. Joseph (1993) provides the following:

> Usually, when we give an interpretation to a patient, we expect some reaction. This can be conscious reflection, reflection on what has been said; but it is still more the unconscious processing or the unconscious establishment of a connection which we would describe as resonance in psychoanalysis.
>
> (p. 1001)

To me, this is akin to what Poland (2017) means when he says that "the becoming as-if-one-with and the separating from are at the heart of both reading and analyzing" (location 361). He goes on to paraphrase Proust's observation that although the reader is involved in a conversation with the author, each of us reads in the midst of our own solitude. Poland argues that what is ultimately assimilated in an analysis occurs within the privacy of the self.

Clinical moments of intimacy

In this section I would like to present various clinical situations that represent, to me, manifestations of what I experienced as intimate moments that occurred in my consulting room. The experience of what is 'intimate' is specific and unique to everyone, so there will be disagreement regarding my choices. The following vignettes represent moments from different analyses. Sometimes it was something that the patient said that made me see something about myself or the world in a new light. Another time it is the privilege of hearing something, revealed for the first time, so honest and so unvarnished in its truth that I have felt humbled by it. And at other times, there can be a feeling of attunement that is so exquisite it is like a perfect chord. Sometimes, it just happens in the space between us, the potential space if you will, and there are no words for it. Inevitably, I will fail to mention any number of excellent examples, but it is hoped that those offered below will generate further conversation.

Resonance

I distinctly remember the morning when Ms. A., a long-time patient, first lay down on my couch. Shortly after we started a twice-weekly psychotherapy together, she began to wish that she could have an analysis. She had come from a chaotic, dysfunctional family with divorces, drugs and pervasive boundary violations. While her history did not suggest that she would be a suitable candidate for analysis, her motivation and intelligence and openness to her emotions did. For various reasons (including a supervisor who had determined from her history that she was unanalyzable and therefore not suitable as a training case), we had postponed this moment for years. At last, I had finished my training and felt confident that she was intact and deeply motivated. When she said one day, "I'm not sure there is more we can do here sitting up; I just wish we could have done analysis", I was able to respond that in fact we were indeed free to begin analysis as my training had been completed and I could make the decision myself. I would argue that this revelation on my part, that I had both finished training and that I had confidence in her, was an intimate moment of enduring consequence for us. The stipulation that a potential analysand must sign an agreement stating that they know their analyst is in training is a highly intrusive overture for an analysis. Interestingly, there is no procedure for the newly minted analyst to announce she has successfully completed her training, so this disclosure was unusual. It signaled that I had achieved some level of expertise and that I had faith in her adequate 'expertise' to undertake an analysis successfully.

Thus, as Ms. A. lay down, I felt a sense of tenderness, as I almost always do when someone lies down for the first time. She sighed, describing what she saw with a sense of wonder, "It's like I am inside looking around and there is a river, and forests, and flowers. It is as if there is so much inside me". I felt an exquisite pleasure in hearing her words, which foretold her experience in her analysis. Despite an extremely difficult childhood with many missteps, she had remained dedicated to creating a better life for herself. In her opening moments on the couch, she reminded me of my own sense of excitement when I began analysis, as well as my recent graduation. I had a feeling of intimate understanding, or perhaps the better word is resonance, with her experience. No words were necessary, although I may have gently, "Mmm-ed" with her. This might also be described as a sort of peak experience, a moment that I felt privileged to share with her.

Familiarity

In this vignette, Mr. W. brought to my attention the difference between intimacy and familiarity which, to his mind, limited the scope of anything we might label as intimate about what he calls 'our relationship'. This was a moment of revelation for me that confirmed my sense that while we have intimate moments with patients, moments that would not take place in any other context, they are also circumscribed by the analytic task, as they should be. Analysis cannot be a long-time substitute for living one's actual life.

Mr. W. had been in analysis for several years. He had been referred to me by his cousin's therapist in another city. Despite the fact that he had difficulty maintaining relationships in his work life as well as his personal life, he took solace in the idea that he was a special person. Part of this view of himself was bolstered by the idea that he was in the most intellectually challenging treatment available, psychoanalysis, rather than a more pedestrian treatment such as cognitive-behavioral therapy. It was important to him to maintain his view that his analyst was a 'teacher', almost in the tradition of gurus, and therefore a superior person as well. At times during sessions, I would be screaming inside my head, "I am not your teacher! I never said that!" In reality, I sat quietly through many hours, wondering how this false edifice could ever be dismantled. One day he came in with a dream that seemed to give him a great deal of peace. In it, he had been in my office where I had been using geometric shapes to explain to him the intricacies of psychoanalysis. This was extremely gratifying to him as he felt I was inducting him into the more arcane intricacies of the process. At the same time, he felt it helped him to understand his feelings. I told him that I needed to see a friend and would have to leave. He asked for a ride but I was initially reluctant to take him, although I eventually consented. We drove to a fast food burger joint in my mid-sized American car. There I met a friend who seemed notably less sophisticated than the way he viewed me at that time. I seemed more 'commonplace'. Still, he felt that he could see more of me and that this dissipated the tension he had felt by seeing me as being on another level from him. I also experienced a new freedom to think my own thoughts in the session with his new de-idealization of me. Additionally, Mr. W. now felt that he had a context for our relationship that doesn't exist in real life. For him, it normalized our relationship because we had a series of ordinary interactions together, e.g. driving in my unremarkable car to a greasy spoon restaurant where I had an unimpressive friend. He found the dream 'personal' in its ordinariness. While friends talk about the commonplace chores of daily life such as grocery lists or what to order at a restaurant, analysts and analysands do not exchange such familiar pleasantries as make up the fabric of daily life. He observed that getting the unconscious to be conscious is indeed a dramatic event that is life changing, but walking the dog and talking to neighbors, i.e. the sharing of simple things, has a kind of intimacy of its own, one that is not possible in the more formal setting of the consulting room. This patient pointed out that while we may have stirring conversations together about the deepest parts of his psyche, conversations that he would have with no one else and that no one else would understand, he still feels a certain tension with me that he believes would be alleviated if he knew more about the quotidian aspects of my day.

Immersed as we are in the world of psychoanalysis, we forget that the people who come to us are not. They come to us by way of a positive referral or even an internet search. For most people, the analytic encounter is a strange situation, unlike any other. As practitioners, we have heard about our analysts from others in our institutes and even if there is an effort to maintain anonymity for the analyst, we know so much about each other just by being in the same profession and usually, the same institute. As analysts, we have been indoctrinated to the mores of our field and already share that knowledge when we begin our training analyses. We talk with our colleagues about our experiences; it is all as familiar to us as meeting a neighbor on a dog walk is to the patient mentioned above. His dream, in which I was willing to teach him about the inner workings of psychoanalysis through these geometric shapes and give him a ride in my car, was so powerful that he felt more comfortable with me afterwards. In fact, in subsequent dreams that week, he found himself empowered to do things he ordinarily would not have been able to do and attributed it to the dream about our interaction. He had an experience of intimacy or familiarity in the dream that he did not experience with me in person and that I do not generally feel with him. Like the patients described by Shane and Shane (1997), I experience him as the patient who uses me as to bolster his self-esteem, rather than an autonomous entity. It is often difficult to accept the roles in which I am placed. Paradoxically, he is the only patient I have ever had who regularly gives me a gift for Christmas. Almost always, it is a book that interests me and frequently it is a book that I have just thought about purchasing. On some level, he intuits a great deal about me that is accurate, far more than I tend to realize.

Reverie

Many years ago, I had a patient, Mr. Y., whose life story was as different from mine as I could imagine. Whereas my family hovered over me, his left him alone in the house for entire summers while they traveled. My parents were parochial in their interests and conversations often revolved around sports whereas his parents were intellectually driven and had a worldly sophistication that conferred on him a citizen of the world status. We grew up in different parts of the country, our educational experiences were disparate, but there was one thing that we shared – our fantasy lives bore an uncanny resemblance to each other (although only I knew this, of course). When Mr. Y. described the way he wanted his apartment to look: a Morris chair, kilim rugs and bookshelves that covered the walls from floor to ceiling, I could almost smell the leather in the chair as he lovingly described it. His idea of a wonderful day was to spend it curled up in front of a fire reading a novel by Edith Wharton and it sounded marvelous but also a bit fey or studied. I never had occasion to say any of this, but from time to time, I would say something that resonated with him and revealed this shared frequency. One morning he was describing his wish to have lived his life fully rather than carefully, so fully that he would be full of knocks and bruises, badges of his brave engagement with the world. This was the counterpart to his fantasy of a contemplative life, enriched by an immersion in literature and libraries. I found myself thinking of the children's book by Marjorie Williams (1922) called *The Velveteen Rabbit*. All the characters in it are stuffed animals and in this passage, the Skin Horse is explaining to a stuffed rabbit how to become Real, not just a stuffed animal.

> "Real isn't how you are made," said the Skin Horse. "It's a thing that happens to you . . . It doesn't happen all at once . . . You become. It takes a long time. That's why it doesn't happen often to people who break easily, or have sharp edges, or who have to be carefully kept. Generally, by the time you are Real, most of your hair has been loved off, and your eyes drop out and you get loose in the joints and very shabby. But these things don't matter at all, because once you are Real you can't be ugly, except to people who don't understand".
>
> (p. 15)

To my surprise, Mr. Y. began to cry. As sometimes happens, the room became hushed and still, save for the sound of his tears. The sound of cars outside seemed as peaceful as bees buzzing on a summer day. I waited. "I was just thinking about that book", he said. "And wondering where my childhood copy of it was, because I want to give it to you when I leave". When he left a few days later, he gave me a paperback version of the book, saying that he could not find his childhood copy. It was a facsimile of the 'real' version that took place on that cold spring afternoon.

It was in our aesthetic sensibility as it existed in our fantasies that Mr. Y. and I connected. I am sure that there were other episodes of resonance with him that I do not recall as vividly; I never explicitly asked, he never said, and I therefore do not know, whether he felt that same meeting of the minds. Our lives remained dissimilar in outward appearance throughout our work together.

Reparations

The feeling of being misunderstood can be quite devastating to any relationship. When a patient is sensitive to slights, enforcing cancelation policies, fee increases and interpretations can all be painful. I had seen Ms. C., a successful but deeply insecure woman, for several months when the following events took place. She was forced to cancel an appointment at the last minute. When I gave her the invoice at the end of the month, she was angry and hurt that I had charged her for it as she was generally so completely reliable. Her face clouded over, her chin wobbled, and she told me that she would pay it, but she wasn't happy about it. At the next session, she told me that she had learned that her insurance did not cover as much of the session costs as she expected and she thought that we would need to discontinue the treatment at the end of the year; we were closing in on the winter holidays. As the session unfolded, she was able to tell me how angry she was that I had charged her for the missed session. When I welcomed her elaboration of her complaints, she was surprised and gratified. Her parents had always asked her to examine what she had done wrong in any given situation that led to her being upset. As we explored the antecedents for her distress, she became increasingly pleased with her ability to express herself without apparently damaging me. The situation changed from one of feeling mistreated to one of Ms. C. feeling a sense of liberation. She laughed and we laughed together when she acknowledged that she didn't really want to end her treatment, she had just wanted to express her anger. In subsequent weeks, she added that my having maintained my policy allowed her to behave similarly at work.

Witnessing

One of the things we do for our patients is to bear witness to the stories of their lives. This is a task that unfolds over the course of many months and sometimes years. While these stories may start out as tidy little narratives, when there is trauma we will not hear the story in a straightforward manner. It is the privilege of hearing 'the most private and unrevealed parts of the person' that binds the analyst and analysand together in a unique relationship that no one else will ever hear in quite the same way. It is this shared history of having the drama unfold painfully that is part of the intimate relationship we share with a patient.

Ms. N. came to see me when she was a bright, young woman in her early 30s. She had had a ten-year analysis with someone in another city, but she was having questions about her choice of career and trouble establishing a permanent love relationship. She badly wanted to have a family. She told me that she had been referred by her older stepbrother. "We had an incestuous relationship when we were growing up, but now he's my best friend", she told me matter-of-factly. I had a brief moment of thinking, "How modern", as I recalled two sisters I knew who lived with their mother and stepfather in a beautiful house with a beautiful butler's pantry, full of mahogany cupboards with panes of glass behind which crystal goblets and highball glasses waited for cocktail parties. There were monogrammed silver ice buckets and cigarette boxes. Their parents were never home and I had found their nonchalant attitude about grownups to be utterly sophisticated. In retrospect, I think they were quite neglected. They were precocious without being mature. All this went through my mind during the initial session. I also wondered if this dismissal of the seriousness of the abuse was the result of a more sophisticated analysis than I could offer at that early point in my career. She had been given my name as well as that of an intimidatingly senior analyst at my institute. Her prior analyst was also more seasoned than me. Nonetheless, Ms. N. had chosen me and so we would proceed as best we could. Her parents had divorced acrimoniously when she was quite young. When her father remarried, she was grateful for the attention that her new, much older, stepbrother showered on her. Over time I learned that he had groomed her for more than just a few sexual encounters. He became a sort of Svengali to her; he had shaped her thoughts about everything from politics to literature to sex. He provided her with sexual materials and had the uncanny ability to make her feel that she had solicited them. All he was doing, he told her, was giving her what she wanted, including sex. His thoughts had penetrated into every crevice of her mind, leaving her with the feeling that he had been the one person in her family who truly cared for her and paid attention to her needs. No wonder I had been thinking about the beautiful neglected sisters in the lonely mansion! Only during our work together did she begin the arduous task of dis-embedding him from her mind. While the actual sexual abuse had not lasted more than a few months, the feeling of having her mind controlled had lingered. There was scarcely any corner of her life that had not been contaminated by his cynical observations. He had given her the feeling that she and he were superior to the rest of the family and in this he had systematically separated her from anyone who she might have told. It took years for the story to emerge and for her relationship with this stepbrother to become suspect in her mind. When she began to see the ways that he had exploited her needy innocence, it was a devastating loss for her. He had been her life guide, her dearest friend, and the ultimate betrayer, though she could not and would not fully accept this. He had also paid more attention to her than anyone else, driven her to school events during which times they would talk over the experiences of her days and her feelings about her friends. He had advised her about everything. She began to wonder how all of this could have taken place in plain sight of both her mother and her father. Had no one thought to wonder why this older brother was spending such an inordinate amount of time with his little sister, giggling and playing wrestling games in the basement? As she began to reexamine his role in her life, she began to question her relationship with her parents. Who were they really? It left her with no one whom she could rely on, except for me, the person to whom she had told the story. Her life improved, she met someone, married and had children, but no one knew the evolution of her story as I did. As she approached termination, she was loath to give up my intimate knowledge of her journey towards freeing herself from her stepbrother. No one in her life would or could ever share that journey with her in the way that I had, even her husband. She had told both her parents about what had happened with her stepbrother. Both expressed regret that this had happened, but neither expressed true grief about their blindness to what was happening. Neither was eager to return to the subject, so Ms. N. and I hold this experience together, an intimate bond that in its uniqueness, mirrors some of the private little world that Ms. N. shared with her stepbrother. It is this world that must be relinquished in order for her to terminate her treatment.

This example is somewhat different from the other moments. It is a series of moments that has resulted in a shared experience that because of its duration makes it unique. There is reality to the fact that she cannot walk that road in the same way with anyone else. Eventually, she must go on to wrestle and digest all of this after termination for the work to reside within her, carried into the rest of her life solo.

Conclusion

As I wrote this chapter, I thought about intimacy as it takes place over time vs. intimacy as it takes place in momentary interludes: transitory, touching and graceful. I think that the latter is how it should take place in a therapy relationship. If the relationship becomes intimate in an ongoing way, something therapeutic is sacrificed. Patients need solitude within the hour, within their minds and within the therapeutic relationship in order to make progress. If efforts are continually made to meet the analyst, to have the feeling of closeness between the two, it may compromise the ability of one or the other of them to think. As Bollas (2006) so eloquently writes, "Rather than separateness and difference leading to emotional distance – as some might assume – such love creates the possibility for a wider range and greater depth of intimacy with the object or other. By perceiving the object's features, the object is loved for itself, not for oneself" (p. 714).

I began this paper by discussing how ideas about intimacy have evolved due to sociological, cultural and psychological influences. Ehrenberg (1974) argued that achieving intimacy requires work on the part of both patient and analyst and that it is essential to a successful treatment outcome. Without the cultural changes that took place in the 1960s that broke down our reverence for hierarchy and authority, could this have become such a compelling argument? As Levenson (1974) articulated so well, as a culture, we no longer believed that any of us, patient and analyst alike, could become neurosis-free. A genuine acceptance of this was required for something authentic, but by no means necessarily intimate, to occur in treatment.

In regards to whether the feeling of intimacy is the same for both analyst and analysand, I think it is different. Analysts have many patients with whom they can share the sorts of conversations that the analysand shares solely with the analyst. As many writers acknowledge, these conversations satisfy our need for thoughtful, emotionally rich interchanges, but we do this with many people over many years. We are more central to our patients' lives than their individual lives are to ours, no matter how invested we may be in them. At various times during the ebb and flow of treatment, we may be pre-occupied with their difficulties, we may spend hours trying to understand the transference and countertransference dynamics that are taking place, and we may empathize with them, but they are ultimately part of a group of patients in our practice. This is all to the good. If any one patient becomes too important to her analyst, it is almost surely an indication of countertransferential issues that may become dangerous to both. In the past, there was a presumption that if an analyst was well enough analyzed, these problems would not occur. If they did, the analyst went back into treatment to work through these issues, such was the faith we held in the ability of psychoanalysis to cleanse us of our internal issues. While consultation and treatment are of inestimable value, I would add that having a full life of his or her own is perhaps the best prophylactic to safeguard analysts from wanting too much from our relationships with our patients.

Epilogue

Chapter 10

The many shapes of intimacy

Lori C. Bohm

The Shape of Water, the 2018 winner of the Oscar for Best Picture, is at once a haunting depiction of loneliness and abuse experienced by societal outsiders, and a fairy tale love story between a mute young woman named Elisa and a fish-man with divine powers. Much of the film takes place in a windowless Cold War era military research laboratory with an eerie, ominous feel. Elisa works there as a night janitor. The fish-man is the especially prized 'asset' for the military, but Colonel Strickland, his handler, treats him brutally and inhumanely, disciplining him with an electric cattle prod. Elisa identifies with the 'asset': they are both unable to speak, they are both lonely, and they have both been severely maltreated. She surreptitiously brings the fish-man boiled eggs, plays jazz for him on a portable record player, teaches him some sign language – and soon, they fall in love. Their connection is poignant and remarkable, ultimately achieving a palpable intimacy.

Indeed, themes of intimacy, and its antithesis, alienation, permeate the film, evoking many of the motifs highlighted in this book. What makes an interpersonal interaction intimate is complex, historically the purview of poets rather than psychoanalysts, notes Salman Akhtarin his evocative, wide-ranging beginning chapter. But in this increasingly high-tech world, in which many relationships start with a swipe on an app, psychoanalysts are ever more aware of the challenges to achieving intimacy. In fact, the 2017 IPA Congress was devoted to the topic. At that conference, Birksted-Breen (Nemas, 2017) observed in her introduction to the panel, "How do we understand intimacy from an intrapsychic model?" that the subject of intimacy is not a simple one even on a descriptive level. A number of the chapters in this book begin with definitions of intimacy, in an effort to delineate the vast territory being explored. What emerges through these many definitions is that achieving intimacy involves both the intrapsychic and the interpersonal: an awareness of and comfort with what is deeply private and internal, along with the relational experience of sharing this private sense of self with an other who acknowledges and understands it (Siamak Movahedi, Chapter 6). As Gurmeet Kanwal (Chapter 4) puts it,

> Intimacy is a circular experience that can either be seen as beginning from one's innermost being and proceeding outward to establish relationships, or it can be seen as proceeding from a relational context that allows the development and experience of one's subjectivity.

Perhaps the capacity for intimacy is really a 'both/and' development. We are born with the need for intimacy and the nascent possibility to experience it. For the fortunate, the capacity for intimacy is nurtured in the interaction between the infant and the mothering person. For some of our patients, the capacity for intimacy only evolves via the therapeutic relationship.

In common parlance, the word 'intimacy' evokes sexuality. To 'be intimate' with another is a euphemistic way of describing a sexual relationship. But sexual relationships may be devoid of intimacy. *The Shape of Water* graphically depicts several permutations of the relationship between sexuality and intimacy. The sex between Colonel Strickland and his wife is mechanical, utilitarian, far from loving and intimate, while the sex between Elisa and the fish-man radiates closeness and intimacy. Thinking about a divergence between intimacy and sexuality brings to mind a patient who preferred what he called "net sex", sexual experience with online partners, to in-person sexual liaisons. What appealed to him about net sex was that he could imagine his partner in whatever way he wanted: she could be 'perfect'– stunningly beautiful and shapely, without blemish, smelling and seeming like the woman of his dreams. And what was even better was that she would not judge him or make demands on him. In other words, he had no interest whatsoever in getting to know and appreciate a real human being, with her own private experience, or in sharing his inner experience with her. Chapter 8 by Todd Essig, Danielle Magaldi and Leora Trub raises related issues that may occur in technology-mediated sexual relationships.

The Shape of Water offers a window into a range of themes in this volume's exploration of intimacy that have not received adequate psychoanalytic consideration previously. One is the intimacy possible through friendship. The film depicts two intimate friendships enjoyed by Elisa, one with her African-American cleaning partner, Zelda, and the other with a gay neighbor, Giles. Despite being mute, it is clear that Elisa has been able to convey her innermost feelings and struggles to these two friends, and they have shared theirs with her. Ultimately, Zelda and Giles risk their lives and their livelihoods to protect, indeed to try to save, Elisa and the fish-man. The movie's subtext dovetails with an important point in Kanwal's chapter on Friendliness, Friendship and Intimacy: friendliness and friendship are key antidotes to xenophobia, which is otherwise depicted in multiple forms in this film's story.

It also becomes clear, as the movie progresses, that Zelda's marriage is anything but intimate. There is no mutual respect, no sense of safety, no trust between these two partners. Yet, Zelda's life has meaning, humor and depth, largely via her intimate friendships. Her character's lot brings to mind several patients who have troubled marriages but healthy intimate friendships. One, a woman from a traumatic background caused by her father's violence, frequently describes intimate conversations with her women friends. Together, they discuss many personal matters, including chronic complaints about their husbands. My heterosexual patient expresses the wish that her closest girlfriend could be her long-term partner, rather than her husband. Similarly, a male patient who feels disconnected from his wife feels most himself with his 'bro' friends with whom he travels and competes in triathlons (c.f. Hirsch, 1997c).

The Shape of Water also briefly touches on another theme in this rich book on intimacy: patriarchy/gender inequality as a barrier to intimacy. One of the many social inequities depicted in the film is that of the 1950s marital structure, in which the man is the boss and the woman, whether or not she is contributing monetarily to the household, is expected to serve the man. The caricatured picture of Colonel Strickland's marriage vividly portrays this pattern. Moreover, Strickland feels that he is entitled to have any woman he wants, and he sexually harasses, and ultimately tries to rape, Elisa, his social subordinate.

In this book, Movahedi's well-researched chapter on barriers to intimacy in Iranian couples explains how traditional gender-role ideology kills any emotional intimacy that may have existed in relationships prior to marriage. A greater percentage of Iranian women than Iranian men obtain college degrees and work in a professional capacity, yet their husbands' expectations, based on patriarchy, do not change. Reading the detailed analysis of this marital dynamic makes it clear that the situation will have long-term negative consequences for Iran, as women choose not to marry or divorce with greater frequency.

Finally, the relationship between Elisa and the 'asset' could be construed as a multicultural, interracial, (and possibly interfaith) 'MII' relationship – after all, it is a romantic relationship between a human being and a scale-covered amphibian! The 'otherness' that could at times characterize how Elisa and the fish-man experience one another is not a focus of this fairy tale. Perhaps the challenges encountered by the couples Bari Smelson-Kanwal treats and describes in Chapter 5 would become evident once the honeymoon phase of the relationship is over. As immigration, technology and access to travel opportunities have made our world more racially, ethnically and religiously interwoven, more and more people find partners who come from a culture, race and/or religion different from their own. The deconstruction of problems interfering with the maintenance of intimacy in these MII relationships is a unique and invaluable contribution to the psychoanalytic literature on intimacy.

Perhaps one reason why *The Shape of Water* won the Academy Award for Best Picture is that it artfully spoke to matters both of the heart and of the social surround that are particularly meaningful to today's audiences. However, another 2018 Best Picture nominee, *The Phantom Thread*, depicts an aspect of intimacy that is not apparent in *The Shape of Water*. *The Phantom Thread*, a deeply affecting film, ultimately induces profound discomfort, as a perverse form of intimacy unfolds. The movie exquisitely details, mostly through its lush close-up photography, the life and work of Reynolds Woodcock, a high fashion designer in 1950s London. He has relationships, but not until a young woman serves him lunch at an inn near his country estate, does he meet his match. On their first date he measures Alma, this couturier's dream of a woman, so that he may create a custom dress for her. Alma becomes his model and muse at the House of Woodcock, as she works to cultivate a relationship with Reynolds in which she truly matters. She does not want to be sent away, like prior models, simply because she is not sufficiently quiet and invisible during breakfast. Shades of the Oedipal color Reynold's behavior: he is deeply attached to his dead mother, whom he believes is watching over him from heaven. She was apparently very demanding and cold, but she taught him his trade and the importance of being fastidious in plying it. It is inferred, but not explicitly stated, that she expected her children to be completely self-sufficient unless they were incapacitated by sickness. In fact, Reynolds's mother's ghost visits him when he is bedridden with an apparent illness. In this state, he becomes entirely physically and emotionally dependent upon Alma as she nurses him back to health. When he begins to recover, he proposes marriage to her. Alma finally understands what she needs to do to create the intimacy she longs for with this difficult, narcissistic man. By finding a way that she can predictably cause Reynolds to fall ill, she assures his need and thus his intimate connection with her.

Yes, intimacy is quite complex and far from always positive. As noted by Salerno (2014) in a review of an earlier book on a related topic, *Intimacies: A New World of Relational Life*, "Intimacy isn't always pretty, and isn't always in the service of personal growth. There can be too much of it. It can be toxic and oppressive, and there are times when it is neither desirable not helpful" (p. 317). For example, Suzanne Benser's chapter on privacy and intimacy in the current volume provides a detailed case presentation in which the reported extreme intimacy between a mother and son prevents him from achieving autonomy. Consequently, he is unable to develop an intimate and sexually healthy relationship with an appropriate romantic partner. Chapter 2 on attachment and intimacy (April Fallon and Rama Rao Gogineni) also sheds light on the possible developmental failures that Benser's patient's analysis ultimately addressed.

While the present volume certainly provides examples of unhealthy or destructive intimacy, its main contributions are in other realms. Specifically, in addition to grappling with what constitutes intimacy, this book delves into three intimacy themes that have previously been neglected or underdeveloped by psychoanalytic writers. They are:

- The developmental prerequisites for intimacy
- Cross-cultural considerations
- New avenues for psychoanalytic exploration about intimacy

The book also adds to the literature offering in-depth exploration of intimacy in the therapeutic relationship, with detailed clinical examples.

Developmental prerequisites for intimacy

> Intimate attachments to other human beings are the hub around which a person's life revolves, not only when he is an infant or toddler, or a school child but through his adolescence and his years of maturity as well, and on into old age.
>
> (Bowlby, 1980, p. 422)

Given the centrality of attachment quality for the achievement of intimacy, Fallon and Gogineni's summary of the literature on attachment in Chapter 2 provides a foundation for much of what follows in this volume. In particular, the authors describe abilities essential to intimacy that develop from the caregiver's responsive interaction with the growing child and characterize those who are securely attached (Cassidy, 2001).

One of these abilities, to feel comfortable with an autonomous self, is addressed not only in Benser's case presentation but also in Akhtar's thoughtful opening chapter. In Akhtar's view, true intimacy involves an appreciation for the separateness of one's intimate partner – of her or his separate thoughts and needs – while simultaneously feeling at one with that partner. This tension between intimacy and autonomy or intimacy and privacy is highlighted throughout the book. Fallon and Goglieri emphasize the importance of the mothering person's ability to allow and enjoy the child's autonomous strivings, while providing a secure base to return to when exploration is complete. This ability, which is evident in people who are securely attached, is not unlike Winnicott's "capacity to be alone" (Winnicott, 1958b). What Winnicott is referring to is the ability of the child (and later, the adult) to be comfortable being on her[1] own ('alone'), while in the company of another (mothering) person and/or alone, in the company of an internalized good object. Comfort with the autonomous self permits the person to be intimate without fearing engulfment by the other (Fallon and Gogineni, Chapter 2).

Two related abilities that are precursors to the development of intimacy are the ability to seek out care and to give care to others. In order for this to happen, the child must have the feeling, from experience with caregivers, that if she asks for help, or indicates a need for help nonverbally, help will be forthcoming. Fallon and Goglieri posit that in intimate relationships, partners feel comfortable to ask for care from one another, and are attuned to the needs of their partners, willingly responding to those needs in an appropriate and non-intrusive fashion. Having been cared for by a person who is sensitively responsive to the child's needs helps the child to be sensitive to others' needs more readily and to be prepared to give care to others.

The final ability necessary for intimacy that develops in the interaction between caregiver and child during the latter stages of attachment development is the ability to negotiate. It is impossible for two people, with their own minds, to be in an intimate relationship without there being disagreements that can best be resolved through negotiation. (The caveat is that there can be intimacy in a relationship characterized by dominance and submission. In that case, the dominant partner always has the final word and the other partner submits. No negotiation is needed. See, for example, *The Story of O* by Pauline Réage, 1965.)

In healthy intimate relationships, being able to negotiate is crucial. If a person has not been able to develop this ability during childhood in interaction with caregivers, intimacy may be hard to achieve. In describing how the analyst works with the patient to increase the person's comfort with intimacy, Levenson notes:

> A relationship of intimacy does not depend on getting over one's fears of intimacy, accepting that they are distortions, allergic responses from the past. Rather, it requires being able to evaluate the other, to negotiate, to compromise, even to fight. Intimacy is not a state of grace; it is an implementational skill and requires mentors and practice.
>
> (Levenson, 1991, p. 516)

If the people who come to us for therapy have not had early relationships that encourage working through differences through negotiation, enactments worked through with the analyst provide new possibilities to develop this ability, which is basic to achieving intimacy.

A paper by Bourdè on "The Fear of Intimacy", presented at the 2017 IPA Congress on Intimacy, notes related developmental achievements that make intimacy possible. They are "differentiation between self and other as well as the capacity to access one's own private inner space" (Masina, 2017, p. 1774). Many authors in the current volume also make reference to these abilities as foundational for intimacy. There may be other developmental prerequisites for intimacy that will become clear over time, but this is an excellent beginning. Patients often come to treatment lacking one or more of these abilities and are able to develop them in psychoanalytic psychotherapy or psychoanalysis. In so doing, their potential for partaking in healthy intimate relationships increases.

Cross-cultural considerations

One of the strengths of this book on intimacy is the rich cross-cultural material included. Several of the authors either grew up in South Asia or have a South Asian spouse, and one grew up in Iran. They are thus able to vividly depict cultural variances of their own, or their partner's, culture as pertains to intimacy. In addition to the information about marital relationships in Iran described above (re: Movahedi's Chapter 6), the reader comes to understand some basic differences between what Indian and American families and intimate friends expect from each other. Akhtar's opening chapter considers not only East vs. West, but Mediterranean and Latin American cultures as well. What is apparent is that psychoanalysis, a Western creation, relies heavily on the cultural and familial customs of Europeans and Americans for theory building, neglecting the variations in, for example, child-rearing practices occurring elsewhere. Eastern (and Mediterranean and Latin American cultures) tend to expect greater filial devotion, expect strong bonds within the extended family and structure their institutions accordingly. For example, mothers in these cultures are given lengthy maternity leaves, as opposed to the six weeks that is normative as a maternity leave in the U.S. (Akhtar, Chapter 1). As David Pauley (Chapter 3) points out in his chapter on intimacy in adolescence, the idea that there is a biologically based drive to separate in adolescence should be called into question, given what is normative in India and other Eastern cultures. In these cultures aunts and uncles have distinctive and important roles in their nieces' and nephews' lives that extend well into young adulthood. And adolescents are expected to participate fully not only in the lives of the members of their families of origin, but also in the lives of extended family members. Sharing beds (or floor space for sleeping) with family members of all ages is typical and unquestioned. Kanwal (Chapter 4) points out that in India male friends hold hands and touch one another in ways that would in the West infer a homosexual relationship. In short, this book offers a broader perspective on its topic by inclusion of culturally relevant positions and expectations about intimacy.

New avenues for psychoanalytic exploration about intimacy

The psychoanalytic investigation of intimacy has generally been limited to two realms: romantic relationships and clinical work (Akhtar, Chapter 1). This book expands the exploration to include friendship and friendliness, cultural comparisons and the impact of technology on intimacy. Essig, Magaldi and Trub's chapter, "Technology, Intimacy and the Simulation of Intimacy" is timely, as it considers how technology affects the possibility for intimacy inside and outside of the consulting room. The authors address the important question, "What is gained and what is lost in screen relations?" Superficially, it seems as if constant connection would provide greater opportunities for intimacy to develop and to be expressed. But Essig et al., argue that screen relations leave users "vaguely unsatisfied", once screen time is over, pointing out that "less is at stake" than in relationships involving physical co-presence. They offer examples that illustrate the way in which attention to screens interferes with family relations, despite the opportunity screens offer to be perennially in touch. In reading the chapter, images of nannies and young mothers pushing strollers while texting or talking on the phone came to mind, accompanied by the sadness I feel for the alert but unattended children being transported. I have come to wonder what the psychological effects will be to young children who live with chronic partial attention from their caregivers. What is ironic is that these same children, when they are older and have their own digital devices, will likely be subject to intrusive oversight by these same parents who will use GPS tracking apps and other digital monitoring of their children's whereabouts and website choices. Digital technology may radically affect how children are raised, including the attention children receive and their opportunities to consolidate a private, intimate space for themselves.

Intimacy in the therapeutic relationship

The chapter by Essig, Magaldi and Trub also provides an excellent segue to an additional important contribution of this volume to the psychoanalytic literature on intimacy. While the book looks broadly at the topic of intimacy in the therapeutic relationship, I will initially consider one aspect, the role that technology is increasingly playing in the provision of psychoanalytic therapy, supervision and teaching. With the availability of digital video platforms like Zoom, FaceTime, Skype, Vsee and others, there has been a push to use these media to provide psychoanalytic education and therapy to people in parts of the world where there are few psychoanalytically trained practitioners. An entire educational program, the China America Psychoanalytic Alliance (CAPA) has successfully been developed to teach Chinese mental health practitioners the theory and practice of psychoanalytic psychotherapy. While the ultimate goal of the program is to train enough Chinese practitioners to enable them to start their own psychoanalytic training institutes in China, at present American psychoanalysts teach, supervise and treat the Chinese students via video platforms. Moreover, given the paucity of well-trained psychoanalytic psychotherapists in China, many of the students in the CAPA program treat patients from other regions in China using these same video platforms. Providing instruction via screens has become common practice universally, with the burgeoning availability of webinars and online courses across the spectrum of academia. Tutoring and clinical supervision, which requires a certain degree of intimacy between student and tutor/supervisor, is still a form of teaching and may be less subject to the subtle considerations that impact intimacy in the psychoanalytic relationship. Hence, our focus will be on "what intimacies are lost?" (Essig *et al.*, Chapter 8) when physical co-presence is not a part of the therapeutic setting.

The IPA's 2017 Congress on Intimacy included a panel entitled "Intimacy and technology: Developing a psychoanalytic dialogue". One of the presenters, John Churcher asked what are "the necessary conditions of the psychoanalytic setting"? He raised two questions about virtual analysis and the essential conditions of the psychoanalytic setting: can confidentiality be preserved? And can virtual presence fully substitute for physical presence? (Bodner, 2017).

If psychoanalytic sessions utilize a HIPAA-compliant video platform, confidentiality can be protected. However, the question of whether virtual presence can fully substitute for physical presence is more complicated. Essig et al. argue that a variety of possibilities for intimacy are lost in analyses conducted in a virtual space. Specifically, the possibility for enactment of a range of therapeutically important fantasies is constricted when analyst and patient do not share the same physical space. The feeling that the therapist is providing a safe, facilitating environment is also curtailed, as patients must provide their own setting for the session and that setting may change with the circumstances of a particular day. Such seemingly trivial items as tissues or paper cups for drinking water, which therapists provide in their physical offices, may hold meaning for patients. Essig et al. suggest that the fantasies that are particularly difficult to enact when the patient is speaking to the therapist on a screen are the destructive ones. Given the challenges to maintaining satisfactory connectivity throughout a virtual session, "screen relations often include a joint effort, a collusion of sorts, to incline treatment towards the attuned and mutual" (Chapter 8). The speakers on the IPA panel on intimacy and technology concur, noting " 'real' as opposed to 'virtual' presence . . . allows for the possibility of giving effect to a phantasy". They add that the real setting "contains the possibility of real action, unlike the virtual setting" (Bodner, 2017, p. 1801). Physical presence allows for the possibility of having an experience in all five senses, including potentially smelling and touching one another. Both Bodner (2017) and Essig et al., (Chapter 8) conclude that what is lost when patient and therapist are not "bodies together" may be more than what is gained by the convenience and expediency of virtual analysis.

In terms of psychoanalyses that take place in the traditional way, in the analyst's office, Christie Platt's Chapter 9 on psychoanalytic intimacy offers a thoughtful exploration of the many facets of intimacy between patient and analyst. She notes that for early models of psychoanalysis, in which analytic neutrality was believed to be essential, as was the notion that the fully analyzed analyst could approach the patient without neurotic impairments, intimacy was seen as something that should not occur in the analytic couple. With the advent of interpersonal and later relational and intersubjective models of psychoanalysis, intimacy between analyst and patient came to be understood by some as crucial to the curative work. From the report on one of the panels at the IPA Congress on Intimacy, entitled, "What does intimacy in the analytic setting mean?", it seems that some classical analysts are still grappling with questions about whether there is intimacy in the analytic situation, and if so, how it can be theoretically conceptualized (Chavis, 2017). For example, the Chair of that panel, Fred Busch, "recognizes analysts who believe intimacy may impair the development of transference" (Chavis, 2017, p. 1775). This conceptualization is in distinct contrast to the work of Ehrenberg (1992) on what she calls "the intimate edge", which involves the analyst's exquisite attention to every aspect of the trajectory of interpersonal experience with a patient. Ehrenberg notes that "[a]ttempting to relate at this point requires ceaseless sensitivity to inner changes in oneself and in the other, as well as to changes at the interface of the interaction" (Ehrenberg, 1992, p. 33). Psychoanalytic exploration of this type is intimate indeed. In *A Meeting of Minds*, an exploration of mutuality in psychoanalysis, Aron (1996) describes Ferenczi's ideas about psychoanalysis: "Ferenczi's search for openness, emotional exchange, closeness and intimacy . . . became incorporated into his psychoanalytic world view" (pp. 162–163). Even as early as the 1920s, a person whose work foreshadowed relational psychoanalysis, understood psychoanalysis as an endeavor involving intimacy between patient and analyst.

Platt's chapter reviews the power, as well as potential dangers, in intimacy between analyst and patient. She notes that the intimacy in the analytic relationship is not perennially felt, but that it often occurs at special, poignant moments in the work, often when the analyst is particularly attuned to her patient. The clinical vignettes she offers beautifully illustrate what others term "moments of meeting" (Stern et al., 1998; Yerushalmi, 2013), instances in which the intimacy between analyst and patient is powerfully felt and is transformational for the patient and often for the analyst as well.

Thomas Ogden, a classically trained psychoanalyst who has been instrumental in describing intersubjectivity and its ubiquitous presence in the analytic relationship, spoke of the intimate exchange between analyst and patient as follows:

> If we, as analysts, are to respond to what is uniquely human about each of our patients, we must develop with the patient an analytic conversation that we could have with no other person in the world. We speak to our spouse or partner . . . to our closest friend, our oldest daughter – to every person with whom we have an intimate relationship – in a way that we would not dream of speaking to anyone else in the world. . . . I am not referring to *what* we say, but to *the way we speak*. . . . [C]reating a unique way of speaking with a patient is not a pre-requisite for analytic work, it is the analytic work.
>
> (Ogden & DiDonna, 2013, p. 629)

In the sense that the analytic field (Ferro & Basile, 2009), or in Ogden's terms, the analytic third (Ogden, 1994) is uniquely created by each analytic couple, the psychoanalytic endeavor is always an intimate one.

Concluding thoughts

In this book we have tried to look widely and thoughtfully at the complex topic of intimacy through a psychoanalytic lens. Intimacy is a word that has both 'secrecy' and 'sociability' as synonyms (Roget's International Thesaurus, 1962), reflecting its dual nature as a private, internal experience and as one that involves deep personal sharing within a close relationship. It is difficult to imagine an aspect of life that is more central to being human than is intimacy. Consequently, psychoanalysis and psychoanalytic psychotherapy are inevitably concerned with intimate matters, whether the therapeutic relationship itself is understood to involve intimacy or not. By expanding the exploration of intimacy to include the consideration of cross-cultural differences, MII relationships, friendship, the impact of technology and the developmental prerequisites for intimacy, this volume makes a unique and valuable contribution to the psychoanalytic literature on intimacy.

Note

1 Rather than describing examples using both gendered pronouns, feminine pronouns will be used throughout. These examples pertain to people of all genders.

References

Abraham, K. (1925). The history of an impostor in the light of psychoanalytical knowledge. In: *Clinical Papers and Essays on Psychoanalysis*, pp. 291–305. New York, NY: Brunner/Mazel, 1955.

Acevedo, B.P., Aron, A., Fisher, H.E., & Brown, L.L. (2012). Neural correlates of long-term intense romantic love. *Social Cognitive and Affective Neuroscience* 7: 145–159.

Ackerley, J. (1956). *My Dog, Tulip*. New York: New York Review Book Classics, 2011.

Adams, G., Anderson, S.L., & Adonu, J.K. (2004). The cultural grounding of closeness and intimacy. In: *The Handbook of Closeness and Intimacy*, eds. D.J. Mashek & A.P. Aron, pp. 321–339. Mahwah, NJ: Lawrence Erlbaum Associates.

Addison, S., & Thomas, V. (2009). Power, privilege and oppression: White therapists working with minority couples. In: *Multicultural Couple Therapy*, eds. M. Rastogi & V. Thomas, pp. 9–27. New York: Sage Publications.

Ahuvia, A.C. (2005). Beyond the extended self: Loved objects and consumers' identity narratives. *Journal of Consumer Research* 32(1): 171–184.

Ainslie, R.C., Harlem, A., Tummala-Narra, P., Barbanel, L., & Ruth, R. (2013). Contemporary psychoanalytic views on the experience of immigration. *Psychoanalytic Psychology* 30(4): 663–679.

Ainsworth, M.D. (1954). Patterns of attachment behavior shown by the infant in interaction with his mother. *Merrill-Palmer Quarterly* 10: 51–58.

Ainsworth, M.D. (1967). *Infancy in Uganda: Infant Care and the Growth of Love*. Baltimore, MD: Johns Hopkins University Press.

Ainsworth, M.D. (1985). Patterns of attachment. *The Clinical Psychologist* 32: 27–29.

Ainsworth, M.D. (1989). Attachments beyond infancy. *American Psychologist* 44: 709–716.

Akhtar, J.N. (1964). *Nazr-e-Butaan*. New Delhi, India: Star Publications.

Akhtar, J.N. (1975). *Pichhale Pehar*. New Delhi, India: Maktaba Jamia.

Akhtar, S. (1989). Narcissistic personality disorder. *Psychiatric Clinics of North America* 12: 505–529.

Akhtar, S. (1990). Concept of interpersonal distance in borderline personality disorder (Letter to Editor). *American Journal of Psychiatry* 147: 2.

Akhtar, S. (1992a). *Broken Structures: Severe Personality Disorders and Their Treatment*. Northvale, NJ: Jason Aronson.

Akhtar, S. (1992b). Tethers, orbits, and invisible fences: Clinical, developmental, sociocultural, and technical aspects of optimal distance. In: *When the Body Speaks: Psychological Meanings in Kinetic Clues*, eds. S. Kramer & S. Akhtar, pp. 21–57. Northvale, NJ: Jason Aronson.

Akhtar, S. (1995). A third individuation: Immigration, identity, and the psychoanalytic process. *Journal of the American Psychoanalytic Association* 43: 1051–1084.

Akhtar, S. (1997). Review of Kurtz, S. (1992): All the mothers are one: Hindu India and the cultural reshaping of psychoanalysis. *Journal of the American Psychoanalytic Association* 45: 1014–1019.

Akhtar, S. (1999). *Immigration and Identity: Turmoil Treatment and Transformation*. Lanham, MD: The Rowman and Littlefield Publishing Group, Inc.

Akhtar, S. (2002). Forgiveness: Origins, dynamics, psychopathology, and clinical relevance. *Psychoanalytic Quarterly* 71: 175–212.

Akhtar, S. (2007). From unmentalized xenophobia to messianic sadism: Some reflections on the phenomenology of prejudice. In: *The Future of Prejudice: Psychoanalysis and the Prevention of Prejudice*, eds. H. Parens, A. Mahfouz, S.W. Twemlow, & D.E. Scharff, pp. 7–19. Lanham, MD: Aronson.

Akhtar, S. (2009a). *The Damaged Core: Origins, Dynamics, Manifestations, and Treatment*. Lanham, MD: Jason Aronson.

Akhtar, S. (2009b). Psychoanalysis and human goodness: Theory. In: *Good Feelings: Psychoanalytic Reflections on Positive Emotions and Attitudes*, ed. S. Akhtar, pp. xxv–xxxv. London: Karnac.

Akhtar, S. (2009c). Psychoanalysis and human goodness: Technique. In: *Good Feelings: Psychoanalytic Reflections on Positive Emotions and Attitudes*, ed. S. Akhtar, pp. 453–467. London: Karnac.

Akhtar, S. (2011). *Immigration and Acculturation: Mourning, Adaptation and the Next Generation*. Lanham, MD: The Rowman and Littlefield Publishing Group, Inc.

Akhtar, S. (2012a). Gratitude. In: *Good Stuff: Generosity, Resilience, Humility, Gratitude, Forgiveness, and Sacrifice*, pp. 53–73. Lanham, MD: Jason Aronson.

Akhtar, S. (2012b). Generosity. In: *Good Stuff: Generosity, Resilience, Humility, Gratitude, Forgiveness, and Sacrifice*, pp. 75–102. Lanham, MD: Jason Aronson.

Akhtar, S. (2013a). *Psychoanalytic Listening: Methods, Limits, and Innovations*. London: Karnac Books.

Akhtar, S. (2013b). Refusing to listen. In: *Psychoanalytic Listening: Methods, Limits, and Innovations*, pp. 125–141. London: Karnac.

Akhtar, S. (2015a). Where is India in my psychoanalytic work? *Psychoanalytic Review* 102: 873–911.

Akhtar, S. (2015b). Some psychoanalytic reflections on the concept of dignity. *American Journal of Psychoanalysis* 75: 244–266.

Akhtar, S. (2015c). Patience. *Psychoanalytic Review* 102: 93–122.

Akhtar, S. (2016). Mistrust, suspiciousness, and paranoia during adulthood. In: *Mistrust: Developmental, Cultural, and Clinical Realms*, ed. S. Akhtar, pp. 41–60. London: Karnac.

Akhtar, S. (2017). The tripod of terrorism. *International Forum of Psychoanalysis* 26(3): 139–159.

Akhtar, S. (2018). Humility. *American Journal of Psychoanalysis* 78.

Akhtar, S., & Brown, J. (2005). Animals in psychiatric symptomatology. In: *The Mental Zoo: Animals in the Human Mind and Its Pathology*, eds. S. Akhtar and V. Volkan, pp. 3–38. Madison, CT: International Universities Press.

Akhtar, S., & Volkan, V. (2005a). *Mental Zoo: Animals in the Human Mind and Its Pathology*. Madison, CT: International Universities Press.

Akhtar, S., & Volkan, V. (2005b). *Cultural Zoo: Animals in the Human Mind and Its Sublimations*. Madison, CT: International Universities Press.

Alperin, R. (2001). Barriers to intimacy: An object relations perspective. *Psychoanalytic Psychology* 18: 137–156.

Alter, A. (2017). *Irresistible: The Rise of Addictive Technology and the Business of Keeping Us Hooked*. New York: Penguin Press.

Ardakanil, N.J., Harehdasht, H.A., & Hajjari, L. (2015). The controversial portrayal of women in Persian proverbs. *English Language and Literature Studies* 5(3): 146–155.

Ariès, P. (1962). *Centuries of Childhood: A Social History of Family Life*, trans. R. Baldick. New York: Vintage.

Aron, L. (1996). *A Meeting of Minds*. Hillsdale, NJ: The Analytic Press.

Aronson, J.K. (Ed.) (2000). *The Use of the Telephone in Psychotherapy*. Northvale, NJ: Aronson.

Bach, S. (1977). On narcissistic state of consciousness. *International Journal of Psychoanalysis* 58: 209–233.

Bach, S. (2006). *Getting from Here to There*. New York: Routledge.

Bakermans-Kranenburg, M., Van Ijzendoorn, M., & Juffer, F. (2003). Less is more: Meta-analyses of sensitivity and attachment interventions in early childhood. *Psychological Bulletin* 129: 195–215. Doi:10.1037/0033-2909.129.2.195

Bakermans-Kranenburg, M.J., & Van Ijzendoorn, M.H. (2016). Attachment, parenting, and genetics. In: *Handbook of Attachment: Theory, Research, and Clinical Applications, Third Edition*, eds. J. Cassidy & P.R. Shaver, pp. 155–179. New York: Guilford Press.

Balint, M. (1953). *Primary Love and Psychoanalytic Technique*. London: Tavistock Publications.

Balint, M. (1968). *Basic Fault: Therapeutic Aspects of Regression*. London: Tavistock Publications.

Balzarini, R.N., Campbell, L., Kohut, T., Holmes, B.M., Lehmiller, J.J., & Harman, J.J. (2017). Perceptions of primary and secondary relationships in polyamory. *PLoS One* 12(5): e0177841. Retrieved from https://doi.org/10.1371/journal.pone.0177841

Bartholomew, K. (1990). Avoidance of intimacy: An attachment perspective. *Journal of Social and Personal Relationships* 7: 147–178.

Baxter, K. (2008). *The Modern Age: Turn-of-the-Century American Culture and the Invention of Adolescence*. Tuscaloosa, AL: University of Alabama Press.

Beck, L.A., Pietromonaco, P.R., DeVito, C.C., Powers, S.I., & Boyle, A.M. (2014). Congruence between spouses' perceptions and observers' ratings of responsiveness: The role of attachment avoidance. *Personality & Social Psychology Bulletin* 40: 164–174. https://doi.org/10.1177/0146167213507779

Behzadi, K. (1994). Interpersonal conflict and emotions in an Iranian cultural practice: Qahr and ashti. *Culture, Medicine and Psychiatry* 18(3): 321–359.

Bekoff, M. (1998). *Animal Play: Evolutionary, Comparative and Ecological Perspectives*. Cambridge: Cambridge University Press.

Bekoff, M., & Jessica, P. (2009). *Wild Justice: The Moral Lives of Animals*. Chicago: University of Chicago Press.

Belsky, J. (1997). Theory testing, effect-size evaluation, and differential susceptibility to rearing influence: The case of mothering and attachment. *Child Development* 64: 598–600. https://doi.org/10.1111/j.1467-8624.1997.tb04221.x

Bendicsen, H. (2013). *The Transformational Self: Attachment and the End of the Adolescent Phase*. London: Karnac Books.

Benedek, T. (1938). Adaptation to reality in early infancy. *Psychoanalysis Quarterly* 7: 200–214.

Bengali, S., & Mostaghim, R. (2016). More women in Iran are forgoing marriage: One reason? The men aren't good enough. *Los Angeles Times*, November 11. Retrieved from http://beta.latimes.com/world/la-fg-iran-unmarried-snap-story.html

Benjamin, J. (2004). Beyond doer and done to: An intersubjective view of thirdness. *Psychoanalytic Quarterly* 73: 5–46.

Bergman, A. (1980). Ours, yours, mine. In: *Rapprochements: The Critical Subphase of Separation-Individuation*, eds. R. Lax, S. Bach, & J.A. Burland, pp. 199–216. New York, NY: Jason Aronson.

Bergman, A. (1999). *Ours, Yours, Mine: Mutuality and the Emergence of the Separate Self.* Northvale, NJ: Jason Aronson.

Bialik, K. (2017). Key facts about race and marriage: 50 years after Loving vs. Virginia. *FactTank News in Numbers-Pew Research Center*, June 12. Retrieved on February 25, 2018, from www.pewresearch.org/fact-tank/2017/06/12/key-facts-about-race-and-marriage-50-years-after-loving-v-virginia/

Binstock, W. (1973). On the two forms of intimacy. *Journal of the American Psychoanalytic Association* 21: 93–107.

Bion, W. (1962). *Learning from Experience*. London: Heinemann Medical Maresfield Library, 1984.

Bion, W. (1967). *Second Thoughts*. London: Heinemann.

Bion, W.R. (1962). The psycho-analytic study of thinking. *International Journal of Psychoanalysis* 43: 306–310.

Bion, W.R. (1970). *Attention and Interpretation*. London: Karnac Books, 1984.

Blos, P. (1967). The second individuation process of adolescence. *Psychoanalytic Study of the Child* 22: 162–186.

Blos, P. (1968). *On Adolescence: A Psychoanalytic Interpretation*. New York: Free Press.

Blos, P. (1979). *The Adolescent Passage: Developmental Issues*. New York: International Universities Press.

Bochner, A. (2017). Heart of the matter: A mini-manifesto for autoethnography. *International Review of Qualitative Research* 10(1): 67–80. DOI: 10.1525/irqr.2017.10.1.67

Bodnar, S. (2004). Remember where you come from: Dissociative process in multicultural individuals. *Psychoanalytic Dialogues* 14(5): 581–603.

Bodner, G. (2017). Panel report, IPA Congress, Buenos Aires 2017: Intimacy and technology: Developing a psychoanalytic dialogue. *International Journal of Psychoanalysis* 98: 1800–1802.

Bolger, N., & Amarel, D. (2007). Effects of social support visibility on adjustment to stress: Experimental evidence. *Journal of Personality and Social Psychology* 92: 458–475.

Bollas, C. (2006). Perceptive identification. *Psychoanalytic Review* 93: 713–717.

Bolognini, S. (2008). *Secret Passages: The Theory and Technique of Interpsychic Relations*, trans. G. Atkinson. New York, NY: Routledge, 2011.

Bolognini, S. (2016). The interpsychic dimension in the psychoanalytic interpretation. *Psychoanalytic Inquiry* 36: 102–111.

Bonovitz, C. (2009). Mixed race and the negotiation of racialized selves: Developing the capacity for internal conflict. *Psychoanalytic Dialogues* 19(4): 426–441.

Bouvet, M. (1958). Technical variations and the concept of distance. *International Journal of Psychoanalysis* 39: 211–221.
Bowen, M. (2004). On the differentiation of the self. In: *Family Therapy in Clinical Practice*, pp. 467–528. New York: Rowman & Littlefield.
Bowlby, J. (1958). The nature of the child's tie to his mother. *International Journal of Psychoanalysis* 39: 350–373.
Bowlby, J. (1969). *Attachment and Loss: Vol. 1: Attachment*. New York: Basic Books.
Bowlby, J. (1973). *Attachment and Loss: Vol. 2: Separation*. New York: Basic Books.
Bowlby, J. (1980). *Attachment and Loss: Vol. 3: Loss, Sadness and Depression*. London: Hogarth Press.
Bowlby, J. (1988). *A Secure Base: Parent–Child Attachment and Healthy Human Development*. New York: Basic Books.
Box, S. (Ed.) (1994). *Crisis at Adolescence: Object Relations Therapy with the Family*. Northvale, NJ: Jason Aronson.
Brabender, V. & Fallon, A. (2013) *Working with Adoptive Parents: Theory, Research and Therapeutic Interventions*. New York: Wiley.
Brahnam, S. (2017). Comparison of in-person and screen-based analysis using communication models: A first step toward the psychoanalysis of telecommunications and its noise. *Psychoanalytic Perspectives* 14(2): 138–158.
Bretherton, I., & Munholland, K.A. (2016). The internal working model construct in light of contemporary neuroimaging research. In: *Handbook of Attachment: Theory, Research, and Clinical Applications, Third Edition*, eds. J. Cassidy & P.R. Shaver, pp. 63–90. New York: Guilford Press.
Brody, E.B. (1978). Intimacy and the fantasy of becoming both sexes. *Journal of the American Academy of Psychoanalysis* 6: 521–531.
Bromberg, P.M. (1996). Standing in the spaces: The multiplicity of self and the psychoanalytic relationship. *Contemporary Psychoanalysis* 32: 509–535.
Bromberg, P.M. (1998). *Standing in the Spaces: Essays on Clinical Process, Trauma and Dissociation*. Hillsdale, NJ: The Analytic Press.
Bromberg, P.M. (2011). *The Shadow of the Tsunami and the Growth of the Relational Mind*. New York; London: Routledge.
Brown, L.J. (2011). *Intersubjective Processes and the Unconscious: An Integration of Freudian, Kleinian and Bionian Perspectives*. New York: Taylor and Francis.
Brown, S., & Christopher, V. (2009). *Play: How It Shapes the Brain, Opens the Imagination, and Invigorates the Soul*. New York: Avery.
Buber, M. (1958). *I and Thou*. New York: Scribner.
Burch, N. (2004). Closeness and intimacy. *British Journal of Psychotherapy* 20: 361–371.
Burghardt, G.M. (2005). *The Genesis of Animal Play: Testing the Limits*. Cambridge, MA: Massachusetts Institute of Technology Press.
Burnet, F.H. (1911). *The Secret Garden*. New York: Dell, 1984.
Burnham, D.L., Gladstone, A.E., & Gibson, R.W. (1969). *Schizophrenia and the Need-Fear Dilemma*. New York, NY: International Universities Press.
Butler, J. (1995). Melancholy gender–refused identification. *Psychoanalytic Dialogues* 5: 165–180.
Cahill, L. (2015). Healing horses: How therapeutic riding lessons can help children with special needs. *The Irish Field*, March 6. Retrieved on December 28, 2017. https://www.theirishfield.ie/healing-horses-how-therapeutic-riding-lessons-can-help-with-special-needs-175861/

Carlino, R. (2011). *Distance Psychoanalysis: The Theory and Practice of Using Communication Technology in the Clinic*. London: Karnac Books.

Casado, E., & Lasen, A. (2014). What is disturbing and why not to disturb: On mobile phones, gender, and privacy within heterosexual intimacy. *Mobile Media & Communication* 2(3): 249–264.

Cashin, S. (2017). *Loving: Interracial Intimacy in America and the Threat to White Supremacy*. Boston: Beacon Press.

Cassidy, J. (2001). Truth, lies, and intimacy: An attachment perspective. *Attachment and Human Development* 3: 121–155.

Cassidy, J. (2016). The nature of the child's ties. In: *Handbook of Attachment: Theory, Research, and Clinical Applications, Third Edition*, eds. J. Cassidy and P.R. Shaver, pp. 3–24. New York: Guilford Press.

Cassidy, J., & Main, M. (1984). The relationship between infant-parent attachment and the ability to tolerate brief separation at six years. *Frontiers of Infant Psychiatry* 2: 132–136.

Cassidy, J., & Shaver, P.R. (Eds.) (2016). *Handbook of Attachment: Theory, Research, and Clinical Applications, Third Edition*. New York: Guilford Press.

Celenza, A. (2015). *Erotic Revelations: Clinical Applications and Perverse Scenarios*. London: Routledge.

Chavis, D.A. (2017). Panel report: IPA Congress Buenos Aires 2017: What does intimacy in the psychoanalytic setting mean? *International Journal of Psychoanalysis* 98: 1775–1778.

Chavooshi, B., Mohammadkhani, P., & Dolatshahee, B. (2017). Telemedicine vs. in-person delivery of intensive short-term dynamic psychotherapy for patients with medically unexplained pain: A 12-month randomized, controlled trial. *Journal of Telemedicine and Telecare* 23(1): 133–141.

Chefetz, R.A., & Bromberg, P.M. (2004). Talking with 'me' and 'not-me': A dialogue. *Contemporary Psychoanalysis* 40(3): 409–464.

Chen, G.M. (1995). Differences in self-disclosure patterns among Americans versus Chinese: A comparative study. *Journal of Cross-Cultural Psychology* 26(1): 84–91.

Chodorow, N. (1978). *The Reproduction of Mothering: Psychoanalysis and the Sociology of Gender*. Berkeley, CA: University of California Press.

Chou, H.G., & Edge, N. (2012). They are happier and having better lives than I am: The impact of using Facebook on perceptions of others' lives. *Cyberpsychology Behavior and Social Networking* 15(2): 117–121.

Ciaramelli, F. (2001). Friendship and desire. *Free Associations* 8(3): 368–389.

Civitarese, G., & Ferro, A. (2015). *The Analytic Field and Its Transformations*. London: Karnac Books.

Colarusso, C.A. (2009). The relentless past. *Psychoanalytic Study of the Child* 64: 320–350.

Common Sense Media. (2016). *Dealing with Devices: The Parent Teen Dynamic [Data file]*. Retrieved on February 4, 2018, from www.commonsensemedia.org/technology-addiction-concern-controversy-and-finding-balance-infographic

Cooper, S.H. (2008). Privacy, reverie, and the analyst's ethical imagination. *Psychoanalytic Quarterly* 77: 1045–1073.

Cooper, S.H. (2014). The things we carry: Finding/creating the object and the analyst's self-reflective participation. *Psychoanalytic Dialogues* 24: 621–636.

Cullen, M. (2011). Mindfulness-based interventions: An emerging phenomenon. *Mindfulness* 2(3): 186–193.

Darooneh, T., Ozgoly, G., Sheikhan, Z., & Nasiri, M. (2017). A Study on the relationship of economic and demographic factors with sexual and marital satisfaction in a sample of Iranian women, 2015–2016. *Journal of Isfahan Medical School* 35(418): 50–56.

Davies, J.M. (2013). My 'enfant terrible' is twenty: A discussion of Slavin's and Gentile's retrospective reconsideration of 'Love in the Afternoon'. *Psychoanalytic Dialogues* 23: 170–179.

Dawkins, R. (2008). *The God Delusion*. Boston, MA: Mariner Books.

de Setton, L.S. (2015). Is there a difference between telephone and in-person sessions? In: *Psychoanalysis Online 2: Impact of Technology on Development, Training, and Therapy*, ed. J. Scharff. London: Karnac Books.

de Wit, M.M., de Vries, S., van der Kamp, J., & Withagen, R. (2017). Affordances and neuroscience: Steps towards a successful marriage. *Neuroscience & Biobehavioral Reviews* 80: 622–629.

Dehghanpisheh, B. (2014). Rise in divorce in Iran linked to shift in status of women. *Reuters World News*, October 22. Retrieved from www.reuters.com/article/us-iran-divorce/rise-in-divorce-in-iran-linked-to-shift-in-status-of-women-idUSKCN0IB0GQ20141022

Demir, M. (2015). *Friendship and Happiness Across the Life-Span and Cultures*. New York, NY: Springer.

Derrida, J. (1993). Politics of friendship. *American Imago* 50(3): 353–339.

DeWolff, M.& Van Ijzendoorn, M. (1997). Sensitivity and attachment: A meta-analysis on parental antecedents of infant attachment. *Child Development*, 68(4), 571–591.

Dicks, H.V. (1967). *Marital Tensions: Clinical Studies Towards a Psychoanalytic Theory of Interaction*. London: Routledge and Kegan Paul.

Diminich, E.D., & Bonanno, G.A. (2014). Faces, feelings, words: Divergence across channels of emotional responding in complicated grief. *Journal of Abnormal Psychology* 123: 350–361.

Dion, K.K., & Dion, K.L. (1993). Individualistic and collectivistic perspectives on gender and the cultural context of love and intimacy. *Journal of Social Issues* 49(3): 53–69.

Donne, J. (1611). A valediction: Forbidding mourning. In: *The Complete Poetry and Selected Prose of John Donne*, ed. C.M. Coffin, p. 38. New York: Modern Library Editions, 2001.

Downes, D. (1966). *The Delinquent Solution: A Study in Sub-Cultural Theory*. London: Palgrave Macmillan.

Durkheim, E. (1893/1960). *The Division of Labor in Society*, trans. G. Simpson. New York: The Free Press.

Durkheim, E. (1897/1951). *Suicide: A Study in Sociology*, trans. J. Spaulding & G. Simpson. New York: The Free Press.

Durkheim, É., Buss, R., Sennett, R., & Riley, A. (1897). *On Suicide*. London: Penguin Books, 1985.

Dykas, M.J., & Cassidy, J. (2011). Attachment and the processing of social information across the life span: Theory and evidence. *Psychological Bulletin* 137: 19–46.

Ehrenberg, D.B. (1974). The intimate edge in therapeutic relatedness. *Contemporary Psychoanalysis* 10: 423–437.

Ehrenberg, D.B. (1992). *The Intimate Edge: Extending the Reach of Psychoanalytic Interaction*. New York, NY: W.W. Norton & Company.

Ehrlich, H.S. (1998). On loneliness, narcissism, and intimacy. *American Journal of Psychoanalysis* 58: 135–162.

Eisnitz, A. (1980). The organization of the self-representation and its influence on pathology. *Psychoanalytic Quarterly* 49: 361–392.
Elston, H. (2018). Behind the veil: Iranian women cast off their hijabs – in pictures. *Guardian*, January 6. Retrieved from www.theguardian.com/artanddesign/gallery/2018/jan/06/behind-the-veil-iranian-women-cast-off-their-hijabs-in-pictures
Erickson, E. (1985). *Childhood and Society*. New York, NY: W.W. Norton & Company.
Erikson, E. (1950a). *Childhood and Reality*. New York, NY: W.W. Norton & Company.
Erikson, E. (1950b). *Childhood and Society, First Edition*. New York, NY: W.W. Norton & Company.
Erikson, E. (1968). *Identity, Youth, and Crisis*. New York, NY: W.W. Norton & Company.
Essig, T. (2012a). Psychoanalysis lost and found-in our culture of simulation and enhancement. *Psychoanalytic Inquiry* 32(5): 438–453.
Essig, T. (2012b). The addiction concept and technology: Diagnosis, metaphor, or something else? A psychodynamic point of view. *Journal of Clinical Psychology* 68(11): 1175–1184.
Essig, T. (2013). The mystery of social media: Talking with ISPSO about 'screen-relations'. *Forbes*. Retrieved on February 4, 2018, from www.forbes.com/sites/toddessig/2013/01/22/the-mystery-of-social-media-talking-with-ispso-about-screen-relations
Essig, T. (2015a). The gains and losses of screen relations: A clinical approach to simulation entrapment and simulation avoidance in a case of excessive internet pornography use. *Contemporary Psychoanalysis* 51(4): 680–703.
Essig, T. (2015b). The 'full training illusion' and the myth of functional equivalence. *The Round Robin* Spring(XXX): 2). Retrieved on January 16, 2018, from http://internationalpsychoanalysis.net/wp-content/uploads/2015/05/RoundRobin2Essig2015FINAL.pages.pdf
Essig, T. (2017). What happens when you can always get what you want: Sex-bots and text therapy. *Forbes*. Retrieved on February 4, 2018, from www.forbes.com/sites/toddessig/2017/08/13/what-happens-when-you-can-always-get-what-you-want-sex-bots-and-text-therapy
Essig, T., & Russell, G.I. (2017). A note from the guest editors. *Psychoanalytic Perspectives* 14(2): 131–137.
Fairbairn, W. (1952). *An Object Relations Theory of Psychoanalysis*. New York, NY: Basic Books.
Fairbairn, W. (1963). Synopsis of an object-relations theory of the personality. *International Journal of Psychoanalysis* 44: 224–225.
Farnam, F., Raisi, F., Janghorbani, M., & Merghati-Khoei, E. (2016). How do Iranian women with sexual problems conceptualize sexuality? A qualitative research. *Nursing Practice Today* 3(3): 107–115.
Feeney, B.C., & Collins, N.L. (2015). Thriving through relationships. *Current Opinion in Psychology* 1: 22–28. https://doi.org/10.1016/j.copsyc.2014.11.001
Feeney, B.C., & Thrush, R.L. (2010). Relationship influences on exploration in adulthood: The characteristics and function of a secure base. *Journal of Personality and Social Psychology* 98: 57–76.
Feeney, B.C., Van Vleet, M., & Jakubiak, B.K. (2015). An attachment theoretical perspective on optimal dependence in close relationships. In: *Attachment Theory and Research: New Directions and Emerging Themes*, eds. J.A. Simpson & W.S. Rholes, pp. 195–233. New York: Guilford Press.
Feeney, B.C., & Woodhouse, S.S. (2016). Caregiving. In: *Handbook of Attachment: Theory, Research, and Clinical Applications, Third Edition*, eds. J. Cassidy & P.R. Shaver, pp. 827–851. New York: Guilford Press.

Feeney, J. Noller, P. & Callan, V. (1994). Attachment style, communication and satisfaction in the early years of marriage. Advances in Personal Relationships. In K. Bartholomew & D. Perlman (Eds.), *Advances in Personal Relationships, Vol. 5. Attachment Processes in Adulthood*, pp. 269–308. London, England: Jessica Kingsley Publishers.

Feeney, J.A. (1994). Attachment style, communication patterns, and satisfaction across the life cycle of marriage. *Personal Relationships* 1(4): 333–348. https://doi.org/10.1111/j.1475-6811.1994.tb00069.x

Feeney, J.A. (1996). Attachment, caregiving, and marital satisfaction. *Personal Relationships* 3: 401–416.

Feeney, J.A. (2016). Adult romantic attachment: Developments in the study of couple relationships. In: *Handbook of Attachment: Theory, Research, and Clinical Applications, Third Edition*, eds. J. Cassidy & P.R. Shaver, pp. 435–463. New York: Guilford Press.

Feldman, M. (2007). Addressing parts of the self. *International Journal of Psychoanalysis* 88: 371–386.

Ferenczi, S. (1928). The elasticity of psychoanalytical technique. In: *Final Contributions to the Problems and Methods of Psychoanalysis*, pp. 87–101. New York, NY: Basic Books, 1955.

Ferenczi, S. (1929). The unwelcome child and his death instinct. *International Journal of Psychoanalysis* 10: 125–129.

Ferenczi, S. (1931). Child-analysis in the analysis of adults. *International Journal of Psychoanalysis* 12: 468–482.

Ferreira, A. (1964). The intimacy need in psychotherapy. *American Journal of Psychoanalysis* 24: 190–194.

Ferro, A., & Basile, R. (eds.) (2009). *The Analytic Field – A Clinical Concept*. London: Karnac.

Fishbane, M.D. (2015). Couple therapy and interpersonal neurobiology. In: *Clinical Handbook of Couple Therapy*, 5th edition, eds. A. Gurman, J. Lebow, & D. Snyder, pp. 681–701. New York: Guilford Press.

Fisher, H.E., Aron, A., Mashek, D., Li, H., & Brown, L.L. (2002). Defining the Brain Systems of Lust, Romantic Attraction, and Attachment. *Archives of Sexual Behavior* 31: 413–419. https://doi.org/10.1023/A:1019888024255

Fonagy, P. (2008). A genuinely developmental theory of sexual enjoyment and its implications for psychoanalytic technique. *Journal of the American Psychoanalytic Association* 56: 11–36.

Fraiberg, S., Adelson, E., & Shapiro, V. (1975). Ghosts in the nursery. *Journal of the American Academy of Child Psychiatry*, 14(3), 387–421.

Fraley, R.C. (2010). *A brief overview of adult attachment theory and research*. Retrieved February 2, 2018, from https://internal.psychology.illinois.edu/~rcfraley/attachment.htm.

Fraley, R.C., & Davis, K.E. (1997). Attachment formation and transfer in young adults' close friendships and romantic relationships. *Personal relationships*, 4(2), 131–144.

Fraley, R., & Shaver, P. (2000). Adult Romantic Attachment: Theoretical Developments, Emerging Controversies, and Unanswered Questions. *Review of General Psychology* 4: 132–154. https://doi.org/10.1037//1089-2680.4.2.132

Fraley, R.C., & Shaver, P.R. (2016). Attachment, loss, and grief: Bowlby's views, new developments, and current controversies. In: *Handbook of Attachment: Theory, Research, and Clinical Applications, Third Edition*, eds. J. Cassidy & P.R. Shaver, pp. 40–62. New York: Guilford Press.

Freud, A. (1965). Normality and pathology in childhood. In: *The Writings of Anna Freud*, Vol. 6, pp. 3–273. New York, NY: International Universities Press.
Freud, E. (Ed.) (1961). *The Letters of Sigmund Freud 1873–1839*, trans. J. Stern & T. Stern. London: Hogarth Press.
Freud, S. (1900). The interpretation of dreams. *Standard Edition* 4–5.
Freud, S. (1905). Three essays on the theory of sexuality. *Standard Edition* 7: 135–243.
Freud, S. (1907). Delusions and Dreams in Jensen's 'Gradiva'. *Standard Edition* 9: 1–96.
Freud, S. (1909a). Analysis of a phobia in a five year old boy. *Standard Edition* 10: 5–149.
Freud, S. (1909b). Notes upon a case of obsessional neurosis. *Standard Edition*, 151–244.
Freud, S. (1910). A special type of object choice made by men. *Standard Edition* 11: 163–175.
Freud, S. (1912). Recommendations to physicians practicing psychoanalysis. *Standard Edition* 12: 109–120.
Freud, S. (1913). Totem and taboo. *Standard Edition* 13: 1–161.
Freud, S. (1914). On narcissism. *Standard Edition* 14: 67–103.
Freud, S. (1915). Instincts and their vicissitudes. *Standard Edition* 14: 117–140.
Freud, S. (1917a). A difficulty in the path of psychoanalysis. *Standard Edition* 17: 137–144.
Freud, S. (1917b). Mourning and melancholia. *Standard Edition* 14: 237–258.
Freud, S. (1918). From the history of an infantile neurosis. *Standard Edition* 17: 1–122.
Freud, S. (1921a). *Group Psychology and the Analysis of the Ego: Standard Edition* 18: 65–143. London: Hogarth.
Freud, S. (1921b). Group psychology and the analysis of the ego. *Standard Edition* 18: 65–144.
Freud, S. (1923). The ego and the id. *Standard Edition* 19: 1–66.
Freud, S. (1924). The dissolution of the Oedipus complex. *Standard Edition* 19: 171–188.
Freud, S. (1927a). Fetishism. *Standard Edition* 21: 152–157.
Freud, S. (1927b). The future of an illusion. *Standard Edition* 21: 5–56.
Freud, S. (1930). Civilization and its discontents. *Standard Edition* 21: 64–145.
Freud, S. (1937). *Analysis Terminable and Interminable: Standard Edition* 23: 216–253. London: Hogarth Press.
Freud, S. (1939). Moses and monotheism. *Standard Edition* 23: 7–137.
Frison, E., & Eggermont, S. (2016). 'Harder, better, faster, stronger': Negative comparison on Facebook and adolescents' life satisfaction are reciprocally related. *Cyberpsychology, Behavior, and Social Networking* 19(3): 158–164.
Galatzer-Levy, R., & Cohler, B. (1990). The developmental psychology of the self and the changing worldview of psychoanalysis. *Annals of Psychoanalysis* 18: 1–44.
Galatzer-Levy, R., & Cohler, B. (1993). *The Essential Other: A Developmental Psychology of the Self.* New York: Basic Books.
Gao, G. (1991). Stability of romantic relationships in China and the United States. In: *Cross-cultural Interpersonal Communication, International and Intercultural Communication Annual, Vol. 15*, eds. S. Ting-Toomey & F. Korzenny, pp. 99–115. Thousand Oaks, CA: Sage Publications.
Gay, P. (1988). *Freud: A Life for Our Time*. New York, NY: W.W. Norton & Company.
Gediman, H. (1985). Impostor, inauthenticity, and feeling fraudulent. *Journal of American Psychoanalytic Association* 39: 911–936.
Geller, S.M., & Greenberg, L.S. (2012). *Therapeutic Presence: A Mindful Approach to Effective Therapy*. Washington, DC: American Psychological Association Publications.
Gentile, J. (2013). From truth or dare to show and tell: Reflections on childhood ritual, play, and the evolution of symbolic life. *Psychoanalytic Dialogues* 23: 150–169.

Gentzler, A.L., Oberhauser, A.M., Westerman, D., & Nadorff, D.K. (2011). College students' use of electronic communication with parents: Links to loneliness, attachment, and relationship quality. *Cyberpsychology, Behavior, and Social Networking* 14(1–2): 71–74.

George, C., Kaplan, N., & Main, M. (1985). *The Adult Attachment Interview*. Unpublished manuscript, University of California at Berkeley. Retrieved on September 30, 2018, from www.psychology.sunysb.edu/attachment/measures/content/aai_interview.pdf

George, C., Kaplan, N., & Main, M. (*1985*). *The Adult Attachment Interview*. Unpublished manuscript, University of California at Berkeley. Retrieved on September 30, 2018, from http://www.psychology.sunysb.edu/attachment/measures/content/aai_interview.pdf

Geser, H. (2006). Is the cell phone undermining the social order? Understanding mobile technology from a sociological perspective. *Knowledge, Technology & Policy* 19(1): 8–18.

Gibson, J.J. (1979). The theory of affordances. In: *The People, Place, and Space Reader*, eds. J. J. Gieseking, W. Mangold, C. Katz, S. Low, & S. Saegert (2014). New York: Routledge.

Gilbert, G. (2010). Retrieved on December 16, 2017 from www.theartsdesk.com/tv/hagai-levy-creator-hbos-treatment?page=0,1

Giddens, A. (1992). *The Transformation of Intimacy*. Stanford, CA: Stanford University Press.

Goldberg, H. (1976). *The Hazards of Being Male: Surviving the Myth of Masculine Privilege*. New York, NY: Nash.

Goluboff, S. (2015). Text to sex: The impact of cell phones on hooking up and sexuality on campus. *Mobile Media & Communication* 4(1): 102–120.

Goodwin, R., & Lee, I. (1994). Taboo topics among Chinese and English friends. *Journal of Cross-Cultural Psychology* 25(3): 325–328.

Greenacre, P. (1951). Respiratory incorporation and the phallic phase. *Psychoanalytic Study of the Child* 6: 180–205.

Greenacre, P. (1960). Further notes on fetishism. *Psychoanalytic Study of the Child* 15: 191–207.

Grinberg, L., & Grinberg, R. (1989). *Psychoanalytic Perspectives on Migration and Exile*. New Haven: Yale University Press.

Guillory, J.E., Hancock, J.T., Woodruff, C., & Keilman, J. (2015). Text messaging reduces analgesic requirements during surgery. *Pain Medicine* 16(4): 667–672.

Gunderson, J. (1985). *Borderline Personality Disorder*. Washington, DC: American Psychiatric Press.

Guntrip, H. (1969). *Schizoid Phenomena, Object Relations and the Self*. New York: International Universities Press.

Harter, S. (2015). *The Construction of the Self: Developmental and Sociocultural Foundations*. New York; London: Guilford Publications.

Hartman, S. (2017). The poetic timestamp of digital erotic objects. *Psychoanalytic Perspectives* 14(2): 159–174.

Hartmann, H. (1960). *Psychoanalysis and Moral Values*. New York: International Universities Press.

Hazen, C., & Shaver, P. (1987). Romantic love conceptualized as an attachment process. *Journal of Personality and Social Psychology* 52(3): 511–524.

Heald, C. (2000). *Intimacy with God*. Colorado Springs, CO: NavPress.

Herzog, J. (1984). Fathers and young children: Fathering daughters and fathering sons. In: *Foundations of Infant Psychiatry*, Vol. II, eds. J.D. Kall, E. Galenson, & R. Tyson, pp. 335–343. New York: Basic Books.

Hirsch, I. (1983). Analytic intimacy and the restoration of nurturance. *American Journal of Psychoanalysis* 43: 325–343.

Hirsch, I. (1997a). Analytic intimacy, analyzability and the vulnerable analyst. *Free Associations* 7: 250–259.

Hirsch, I. (1997b). The integration of the interpersonal school into the psychoanalytic mainstream: A review essay on a 'Meeting of Minds: Mutuality in Psychoanalysis' by Lewis Aron. *Contemporary Psychoanalysis* 33: 656–668.

Hirsch, I. (1997c). On men's preference for men. *Gender and Psychoanalysis* 2(4): 469–486.

Hitchens, C. (2007). *God Is Not Great*. New York: Twelve.

Hjorth, L., & Lim, S. (2012). Mobile intimacy in an age of affective mobile media. *Feminist Media Studies* 12(4): 477–484.

Hobbs, M., Owen, S., & Gerber, L. (2017). Liquid love? Dating apps, sex, relationships and the digital transformation of intimacy. *Journal of Sociology* 53(2): 271–284.

Hofer, B.K., & Moore, A.S. (2010). *The iConnected Parent: Staying Close to Your Kids in College (and Beyond) While Letting Them Grow up*. New York, NY: Free Press.

Hoffman, I.Z. (1998). *Ritual and Spontaneity in the Psychoanalytic Process: A Dialectical – Constructivist View*. Hillsdale, NJ: The Analytic Press.

Horner, A. (1986). *Being and Loving*. Northvale, NJ: Jason Aronson.

Howe, D.W. (2007). *What hath God wrought: The transformation of America, 1815–1848*. New York: Oxford University Press.

Howes, C., & Spieker, S. (2016). Attachment relationships in the context of multiple caregivers. In: *Handbook of Attachment: Theory, Research, and Clinical Applications*, eds. J. Cassidy & P. Shaver. New York: The Guilford Press.

Hsu, F.L.K. (1985). The self in cross-cultural perspective. In: *Culture and Self: Asian and Western Perspectives*, eds. A.J. Marsella, G. DeVos & F.L.K. Hsu, pp. 24–55. London: Tavistock Publications.

Hudson, N.W., & Fraley, R.C. (2017). Adult attachment and perceptions of closeness: Attachment and closeness perceptions. *Personal Relationships* 24: 17–26.

Iida, M., Seidman, G., Shrout, P.E., Fujita, K., & Bolger, N. (2008). Modeling support provision in intimate relationships. *Journal of Personality and Social Psychology* 94: 460–478.

Ingram, D.H. (1986). Remarks on intimacy and the fear of commitment. *American Journal of Psychoanalysis* 46: 76–79.

Intimacy. *Dictionary.com*. Retrieved on January 26, 2018, from www.dictionary.com/-browse/intimacy

Intimacy: Origin and Meaning of Intimacy by Online Etymology Dictionary. Retrieved on February 2, 2018, from www.etymonline.com/word/intimacy

Intimacy. Random House. (2018). Retrieved from https://www.dictionary.com/browse/intimacy?s=t

Intimus. *Wiktionary*. Retrieved on February 2, 2018, from https://en.wiktionary.org/wiki/intimus

Jakes, T.D. (2013). *Intimacy with God*. Ada, MI: Bethany House Publishing.

Jamieson, L. (1998). *Intimacy: Personal Relationships in Modern Societies*. Cambridge; Oxford: Polity Press; Blackwell.

Javidan, M., & Dastmalchian, A. (2003). Culture and leadership in Iran: The land of individual achievers, strong family ties, and powerful elite. *Academy of Management Executive* 17(4): 127–142.

Jones, J.D., Cassidy, J., & Shaver, P.R. (2015). Adult attachment style and parenting. In: *Attachment Theory and Research: New Directions and Emerging Themes*, eds. J.A. Simpson & W.S. Rholes, pp. 234–260. New York, NY: Guilford Press.

Joseph, B. (1989). *Psychic Equilibrium and Psychic Change: Selected Papers of Betty Joseph*, eds. M. Feldman & E.B. Spillius. London: Tavistock; Routledge.

Joseph, B. (1993). A factor that counteracts psychic change: No resonance. *Psyche-Z Psychoanalysis* 47: 997–1012.

Joyce, A. (2014). Many kids think parents are too distracted, according to annual survey by Highlights for Children Magazine. *The Washington Post*, October 9. Retrieved on February 4, 2018, from www.washingtonpost.com/news/parenting/wp/2014/10/09/many-kids-think-parents-are-too-distracted-according-to-annual-survey-by-highlights-for-children-magazine/

Kafka, J. (1989). *Multiple Realities in Clinical Practice*. New Haven, CT: Yale University Press.

Kantrowitz, J.L. (2009). Privacy and disclosure in psychoanalysis. *Journal of the American Psychoanalytic Association* 57: 787–806.

Kanwal, G. (2017). 'Benevolent transformation' and the centrality of idealization dynamics in Indian culture. *Psychoanalytic Discourse* 3(February): 11–19. Retrieved from www.psychoanalyticdiscourse.com/index.php/psad/article/view/41

Kaplan, H. (1990). Sex, intimacy, and the aging process. *Journal of American Academy of Psychoanalysis and Dynamic Psychiatry* 18: 185–205.

Keating, T. (2009). *Intimacy with God*. New York: Crossroad Publishing Company.

Kernberg, O. (1970). A psychoanalytic classification of character pathology. *Journal of the American Psychoanalytic Association* 18: 800–822.

Kernberg, O. (1975). *Borderline Conditions and Pathological Narcissism*. New York, NY: Jason Aronson Press.

Kernberg, O. (1984). *Severe Personality Disorders: Psychotherapeutic Strategies*. New Haven, CT: Yale University Press.

Kernberg, O. (1992). *Aggression in Personality Disorders and Perversions*. New Haven, CT: Yale University Press.

Kernberg, O. (1995). *Love Relations: Normality and Pathology*. New Haven, CT: Yale University Press.

Khalifian, C.E., & Barry, R.A. (2016). Trust, attachment, and mindfulness influence intimacy and disengagement during newlyweds' discussions of relationship transgressions. *Journal of Family Psychology* 30: 592–601.

Khan, M. (1979). *Alienation in Perversions*. New York, NY: International Universities Press.

Khan, M. (1983). On lying fallow. In: *Hidden Selves: Between Theory and Practice in Psychoanalysis*, pp. 183–188. New York: International Universities Press.

Khoei, E.M., & Richters, J. (2008). Concepts of sexuality and health among Iranian women in Australia. *Australian Family Physician* 37(3): 190–192.

Khoei, E.M., Whelan, A., & Cohen, J. (2008). *Sharing Beliefs: What Sexuality Means to Muslim Iranian Women Living in Australia*, pp. 237–248. Retrieved on April 23, 2008, from https://doi.org/10.1080/13691050701740039

Kia, M. (2016). Indian friends, Iranian selves, Persianate modern. *Comparative Studies of South Asia, Africa and the Middle East* 36(3): 398–417.

Killian, K. (2002). Dominant and marginalized discourses in interracial couples' narratives: Implications for family therapists. *Family Process* 41(4): 603–618.

Killian, K. (2017). *Interracial Couples, Intimacy and Therapy: Crossing Racial Borders*. New York: Columbia University Press.

Kimmel, M. (2008). *Guyland*. New York: Harper Collins.

Kinsey, A., Pomeroy, W., & Martin, C. (1948a). *Sexual Behavior in the Human Male*. Philadelphia, PA: W.B. Saunders.

Kinsey, A., Pomeroy, W., & Martin, C. (1948b). *Sexual Behavior in the Human Female*. Philadelphia, PA: W.B. Saunders.

Klein, M. (1935). A contribution to the psychogenesis of manic depressive states. In: *Love, Guilt and Reparation and Other Works – 1921–1945*, pp. 262–289. New York, NY: Free Press, 1975.

Klein, M. (1946). Notes on some schizoid mechanisms. *International Journal of Psychoanalysis* 27: 99–110.

Kobak, R., Zajac, K., & Madsen, S.D. (2016). Attachment disruptions, reparative processes, and psychopathology: Theoretical and clinical implications. In: *Handbook of Attachment: Theory, Research, and Clinical Applications, Third Edition*, eds. J. Cassidy & P.R. Shaver, pp. 25–39. New York: Guilford Press.

Kohut, H. (1971). *Analysis of the Self*. New York: International Universities Press.

Kohut, H. (1977). *The Restoration of the Self*. New York: International Universities Press.

Kramer, S. (1996). The development of intimacy and its relationship with the ability to have friends. In: *Intimacy and Infidelity: Separation-Individuation Perspectives*, eds. S. Akhtar and S. Kramer, pp. 1–18. Northvale, NJ: Jason Aronson.

Krayer, A., Ingledew, D.K., & Iphofen, R. (2008). Social comparison and body image in adolescence: A grounded theory approach. *Health Education Research* 23(5): 892–903.

Kretschmer, E. (1925). *Physique and Character*, trans. W.J.H. Sprott. New York: Harcourt-Brace.

Kristeva, J. (1994). *Strangers to Ourselves*. New York: Columbia University Press.

Kurtz, S. (1992). *All The Mothers Are One: Hindu India and the Cultural Re-shaping of Psychoanalysis*. New York: Columbia University Press.

Kurzweil, R. (2001). *The Law of Accelerating Returns*. Retrieved on January 14, 2018, from www.baxtek.com/products/wireless/files/law-of-accelerating-returns.pdf

Laplanche, J. (1995). Seduction, persecution, revelation. *International Journal of Psycho-Analysis* 76: 663–682.

Lasch, C. (1979). *The Culture of Narcissism: American Life in an Age of Diminishing Expectations*. New York, NY: W.W. Norton & Company.

Lee-Won, R.J., Herzog, L., & Park, S.G. (2015). Hooked on Facebook: The role of social anxiety and need for social assurance in problematic use of Facebook. *Cyberpsychology, Behavior and Social Networking* 18(10): 567–574.

Lemma, A. (2017). *The Digital Age on the Couch: Psychoanalytic Practice and New Media*. Washington, DC: Taylor & Francis.

Levenson, E.A. (1974). Changing concepts of intimacy in psychoanalytic practice. *Contemporary Psychoanalysis* 10(3): 359–369.

Levenson, E.A. (1991). Standoffs, impasses and stalemates. *Contemporary Psychoanalysis* 27: 511–517.

Levenson, E.A. (1996). Aspects of self-revelation and self-disclosure. *Contemporary Psychoanalysis* 32(2): 237–248.

Levenson, R. (1984). Intimacy, autonomy, and gender: Developmental differences and their reflection in adult relationships. *Journal of the American Academy of Psychoanalysis* 12: 529–544.

Lévi-Strauss, C. ([1951] 1963). *Structural Anthropology*, trans. C. Jacobson & B. Schoepf. New York: Basic Books.

Levy, R. (2017). Intimacy: The drama and beauty of encountering the other. *International Journal of Psycho-Analysis* 98(3): 877–894.

Lifton, R.J. (1971). Protean man. *Archives of General Psychiatry* 24: 298–304.

Lipka, M., & Gecewicz, C. (2017). More Americans say they're spiritual but not religious. *FactTank Pew Research Analysis*, September 6. Retrieved on February 25, 2018, from www.pewresearch.org/fact-tank/2017/09/06/more-americans-now-say-theyre-spiritual-but-not-religious/

Livingston, G. (2017). Among U.S. cohabitators 18% have a partner of a different ethnicity. 46% Asians are living with a person of a different race or ethnicity. *Factank: Pew Research Center*, June 8. Retrieved on March 2, 2018, from www.pewresearch.org/fact-tank/2017/06/08/among-u-s-cohabiters-18-have-a-partner-of-a-different-race-or-ethnicity/

Livingston, G., & Brown, A. (2017). Intermarriage in the U.S. 50 years after Loving vs. Virginia. *Pew Research Center*. Retrieved on February 25, 2018, from www.pewsocialtrends.org/2017/05/18/intermarriage-in-the-u-s-50-years-after-loving-v-virginia/

Loewald, H.W. (1979). The waning of the Oedipus complex. *Journal of the American Psychoanalytic Association* 27: 751–775.

Lombard, M., & Jones, M.T. (2013). Telepresence and sexuality: A review and a call to scholars. *Human Technology: An Interdisciplinary Journal on Humans in ICT Environments* 9(1): 22–55.

Lucassen N., Tharner, A., Van Ijzendoorn, M., Bakermans-Kranenburg, M., Volling B,. Verhulst, F., Lambregtse-Van den Berg, M., & Tiemeier, H. (2011). The association between paternal sensitivity and infant–father attachment security: A meta-analysis of three decades of research. *Journal of Family Psychology*, *25*(6), 986–992. doi:10.1037/a0025855.

Lup, K., Trub, L., & Rosenthal, L. (2015). Instagram #instasad?: Exploring associations among Instagram use, depressive symptoms, negative social comparison, and strangers followed. *Cyberpsychology, Behavior, and Social Networking* 18(5): 247–252.

Magaldi, D., Appel, R., & Berler, M. (in press). Adolescence and social media use. In: *The Encyclopedia of Child and Adolescent Development*, eds. S. Hupp & J. Jewell. Hoboken, NJ: Wiley-Blackwell.

Magaldi-Dopman, D., & Park-Taylor, J. (2010). Sacred adolescence: Practical suggestions for psychologists working with adolescents' religious and spiritual identity. *Professional Psychology: Research and Practice* 41(5): 382–390.

Mahler, M.S., Pine, F., & Bergman, A. (1975). *The Psychological Birth of the Human Infant: Symbiosis and Individuation*. New York, NY: Basic Books.

Main, M., & Solomon, J. (1990). Procedures for identifying infants as disorganized/disoriented during the Ainsworth Strange Situation. In: *The John D. and Catherine T. MacArthur Foundation series on mental health and development. Attachment in the preschool years: Theory, research, and intervention*, eds. M.T. Greenberg, D. Cicchetti, & E.M. Cummings, eds., pp. 121–160. Chicago, IL: University of Chicago Press.

Majolo, B., Kaye, A., Brumpton, R., Garratt, R., Hall, K., & Wilson, N. (2006). Human friendship favours cooperation in the Iterated Prisoner's Dilemma. *Behavior* 143(11): 1383–1395.

Manago, A.M., Taylor, T., & Greenfield, P.M. (2012). Me and my 400 friends: The anatomy of college students' Facebook networks, their communication patterns, and well-being. *Developmental Psychology* 48(2): 369–380.

Margolis, G.J. (1966). Secrecy and identity. *International Journal of Psychoanalysis* 47: 517–522.

Marshall, T. (2008). Cultural differences in intimacy: The Influence of gender-role ideology and individualism-collectivism. *Journal of Social and Personal Relationships* 25(1): 143–168.

Marvin, R., Britner, P., & Russell, B. (2016). Normative Development: The Ontogeny of Attachment in Childhood, In: *Handbook of attachment: Theory, Research, and Clinical Applications*, eds. J. Cassidy & P. Shaver. New York: The Guilford Press.

Masina, L. (2017). Panel report: IPA Congress Buenos Aires 2017: Fear of intimacy: The pervert's uncanny false intimacy. *International Journal of Psychoanalysis* 98: 1773–1775.

Mayseless, O., & Scharf, M. (2007). Adolescents' attachment representations and their capacity for intimacy in close relationships. *Journal of Research on Adolescence* 17: 23–50.

McDaniel, B.T., & Radesky, J.S. (2018). Technoference: Parent distraction with technology and associations with child behavior problems. *Child Development* 89(1): 100–109.

McKnight, A. (2016). *The Changing Narratives of Intimacy in the Ann Lander's Advice Column*. Doctoral Dissertation, Boston Graduate School of Psychoanalysis.

McKnight, A., & Movahedi, S. (2017). *The Psychoanalytic Significance of the 'Currency of Intimacy' Within the Evolving Cultural Systems of Emotional Exchange*. Paper presented at The IPA Buenos Aires Congress, in July 25–29.

Meins, E., Fernyhough, C., de Rosnay, M., Arnott, B., Leekam, S.R., & Turner, M. (2012). Mind-mindedness as a multidimensional construct: Appropriate and nonattuned mind-related comments independently predict infant–mother attachment in a socially diverse sample. *Infancy*, 17(4), 393–415.

Meissner, W. (1984). *Psychoanalysis and Religious Experience*. New Haven, CT: Yale University Press.

Meissner, W. (2001). So help me God! Do I help God or does God help me? In: *Does God Help? Developmental and Clinical Aspects of Religious Belief*, eds. S. Akhtar & H. Parens, pp. 74–126. Northvale, NJ: Jason Aronson.

Melges, F.T., & Swartz, M.S. (1989). Oscillations of attachment in borderline personality disorder. *American Journal of Psychiatry* 146: 1115–1120.

Meltzer, D. (1971). Sincerity: A study in the atmosphere of the human relations. In: *Sincerity and Other Works: Collected papers of Donald Meltzer*, ed. A. Hahn, pp. 184–284. London: Karnac Books, 1994.

Mihailidis, P. (2014). A tethered generation: Exploring the role of mobile phones in the daily life of young people. *Mobile Media and Communication* 2(1): 58–72.

Mikulincer, M., & Shaver, P.R. (2016). Adult attachment and emotion regulation. In: *Handbook of Attachment: Theory, Research, and Clinical Applications, Third Edition*, eds. J. Cassidy & P.R. Shaver, pp. 507–533. New York: Guilford Press.

Miller, J.F. (2013). *The Triumphant Victim: A Psychoanalytical Perspective on Sadomasochism and Perverse Thinking*. London: Karnac Books.

Minturn, L., & Hitchcock, J.T. (1966). *The Rajputs of Khalapur, India*. New York: John Wiley & Sons.

Mish, F.C. (Ed.) (1998). *Merriam Webster's Collegiate Dictionary, Tenth Edition*. Springfield, MA: Merriam Webster Press.

Mishne, J. (2002). *Multiculturalism and the Therapeutic Process*. New York: Guilford Press.

Mitchell, S. (2002). *Can Love Last? The Fate of Romance over Time*. New York: W.W. Norton and Company.

Mohammad-Alizadeh-Charandabi, S., Mirghafourvand, M., Asghari-Jafarabadi, M., Tavananezhad, N., & Karkhaneh, M. (2014). Modeling of socio-demographic predictors of sexual function in women of reproductive age. *Journal of the Mazandaran University of Medical* Science 23(110): 238–242 (Persian).

Moshtagh, N. (2017). *Femininity and Women's Struggle for Their Inner Voice: A Focused Group Study*. Unpublished Farsi Manuscript. Tehran, Iran: HamAva Institute of Psychotherapy.

Movahedi, S. (1996). Metalinguistic analysis of therapeutic discourse. *Journal of the American Psychoanalytic Association* 44(3): 837–862.

Movahedi, S., & Moshtagh, N. (2018). Persian tales on the couch: Notes on folktales as the mirror of the contemporary cultural struggles with gender and sexuality. *International Forum of Psychoanalysis* (Forthcoming).

Murphy, C. (2011). Unique therapy uses horses to help children. *Farm Ireland*, July 6. Retrieved on December 28, 2017.

Murphy, C. (2015). Interfaith marriage is common in the U.S. particularly among the recently wed. *FactTank – Pew Research Center*, June 2. Retrieved on February 25, 2018, from www.pewresearch.org/fact-tank/2015/06/02/interfaith-marriage/

Nasehi, A.A., Raisi, F., Ghaeli, P., Amini, M., Yahyavi, S.T., Arabkheradmand, J., Faghihzadeh, S., Abbasi, Z., & Abdi, F. (2017). Prevalence of sexual dysfunction among general population of Iran: A systematic review. *Iran Journal of Psychiatry and Behavioral Science*. Retrieved on June 20, 2017, from http://ijpsychiatrybs.com/en/articles/7643.html/ doi:10.5812/ijpbs.7643

Nemas, C. (2017). Panel report: IPA congress Buenos Aires 2017: How do we understand intimacy from an intrapsychic model: Where is the unconscious in the concept of intimacy? *International Journal of Psychoanalysis* 98: 1763–1766.

Neri, D.J. (2018). The need for nuance in the tech use debate: A conversation with Amy Orben. *Behavioral Scientist*, January 1. Retrieved on February 4, 2018, from http://behavioralscientist.org/need-nuance-conversation-amy-orben/

Nicholi, A. (2002). *The Question of God: C.S. Lewis and Sigmund Freud Debate God, Love, Sex, and the Meaning of Life*. New York: Free Press.

Nin, A. (1966). *In Favor of the Sensitive Man, and Other Essays*. Boston, MA: Mariner Books.

Nosek, L. (2009). Body and infinite: Notes for a theory of genitality. *Revista Brasiliera de Psicanalise* 43: 139–151.

Nunberg, H., & Federn, P. (1962). *Minutes of the Vienna Psychoanalytic Society, Vol I: 1906–1908*. New York: International Universities Press.

Oberto, R. (2017). *Intimacy with God*. New York: Opened Heart Publications.

Ogden, T.H. (1991). Some theoretical comments on personal isolation. *Psychoanalytic Dialogues* 1: 377–390.

Ogden, T.H. (1994). The analytic field: Working with intersubjective clinical facts. *International Journal of Psychoanalysis* 75: 3–19.

Ogden, T.H. (1996). Reconsidering three aspects of psychoanalytic technique. *International Journal of Psychoanalysis* 77: 883–889.

Ogden, T.H. (1997). Reverie and interpretation. *Psychoanalytic Quarterly* 66: 567–595.

Ogden, T.H. (2004). This art of psychoanalysis: Dreaming undreamt dreams and interrupted cries. *International Journal of Psycho-Analysis* 85(4): 857–877.

Ogden, T., & DiDonna, L. (2013). Thomas Ogden in conversation with Luca DiDonna. *Rivista di Psicoanalisi* 59(3): 625–641.

Ohadi, J., Brown, B., Trub, L., & Rosenthal, L. (2017). I just text to say I love you: Partner similarity in texting and relationship satisfaction. *Computers in Human Behavior* 78: 126–132.

Orbach, S. (2007). Separated attachments and sexual aliveness: How changing attachment patterns can enhance intimacy. *Attachment: New Directions in Psychotherapy and Relational Psychoanalysis* 1: 8–17.

O'Reilly, T. (2017). *WTF? What's the Future and Why It's up To Us*. New York, NY: HarperCollins.

Ostow, M. (1995). *The Ultimate Intimacy: Psychoanalysis and Jewish Mysticism*. London: Karnac.

Overall, N.C., Fletcher, G.J.O., Simpson, J.A., & Fillo, J. (2015). Attachment insecurity, biased perceptions of romantic partners' negative emotions, and hostile relationship behavior. *Journal of Personality and Social Psychology* 108: 730–749. https://doi.org/10.1037/a0038987

Paris, J. (1985). Boundary and intimacy. *Journal of the American Academy of Psychoanalysis* 13: 505–510.

Parkhurst, C. (2004). *The Dogs of Babel*. Boston, MA: Back Bay Books.

Paul, R. (2005). Anthropology. In: *Textbook of Psychoanalysis*, eds. E.S. Person, A.M. Cooper, & G.O. Gabbard, pp. 479–490. Washington, DC: American Psychiatric Publishing.

Pellis, S.M., Pellis, V.C., & Bell, H.C. (2010). The function of play in the development of the social brain. *American Journal of Play* Winter: 278–296.

Pettigrew, J. (2009). Text messaging and connectedness within close interpersonal relationships. *Marriage & Family Review* 45(6–8): 697–716.

Pietromonaco, P.R., & Beck, L.A. (2015). Attachment processes in adult romantic relationships. In: *APA Handbook of Personality and Social Psychology, Volume 3: Interpersonal Relations*, eds. M. Mikulincer, P.R. Shaver, J.A. Simpson, & J.F. Dovidio, pp. 33–64. Washington, DC: American Psychological Association.

Pizer, B. (2014). A clinical exploration of moving anger forward: Intimacy, anger, and creative freedom. *Psychoanalytic Dialogues* 24(1): 14–28.

Platt, C. (2017). Death of pet. In: *Bereavement: Personal Experiences and Clinical Reflections*, eds. S. Akhtar & G.S. Kanwal, pp. 143–166. London: Karnac.

Plowman, L., McPake, J., & Stephen, C. (2010). The technologisation of childhood? Young children and technology in the home. *Children & Society* 24(1): 63–74.

Poland, W. (2017). *Intimacy and Separateness in Psychoanalysis*. London: Routledge.

Purser, G.S. (2007). Subjectivity or intimacy? The chicken or the egg? What comes first? *Psychotherapy and Relational Psychoanaly*sis 1(3): 294–296.

Quiroz, P.A. (2013). From finding the perfect love online to satellite dating and 'loving-the-one-you're near': A look at Grindr, Skout, Plenty of Fish, Meet Moi, Zoosk and Assisted Serendipity. *Humanity & Society* 37(2): 181–185.

Radesky, J.S., Kistin, C.J., Zuckerman, B., Nitzberg, K., Gross, J., Kaplan-Sanoff, M., & Silverstein, M. (2014). Patterns of mobile device use by caregivers and children during meals in fast food restaurants. *Pediatrics* 133(4): 843–849.

Radomisli, M. (1968). Love, friendship and aim-inhibited aggression. *Psychoanalytic Review* 55(1): 57–61.

Rangell, L. (1963). On friendship. *Journal of the American Psychoanalytic Association* 11: 3–54.

Ranney, J.D., & Troop-Gordon, W. (2012). Computer-mediated communication with distant friends: Relations with adjustment during students' first semester in college. *Journal of Educational Psychology* 104(3): 848–861.

Rao, D. (2005). Manifestations of God in India: A transference patheon. In: *Freud Along the Ganges: Psychoanalytic Reflections on the People and Culture of India*, ed. Salman Akhtar, pp. 271–308. New York, NY: The Other Press.

Random House. (2018). *Intimacy*. Retrieved from www.dictionary.com/browse/intimacy?s=t

Réage, P. (1965). *The Story of O*. New York: Ballantine Books.

Reich, W. (1933). *Character Analysis*. New York: Farrar, Strauss and Giroux, 1972.

Rellahan, M. (2017). Equine therapy helps Chesco inmates. *Philadelphia Inquirer*, B-4, December 26.

Ren, D., Arriaga, X.B., & Mahan, E.R. (2017). Attachment insecurity and perceived importance of relational features. *Journal of Social and Personal Relationships* 34: 446–466.

Richards, A.K., & Spira, L. (2003). On being lonely: Fear of one's own aggression as an impediment to intimacy. *Psychoanalytic Quarterly* 72: 257–374.

Rizzuto, A.M. (1979). *The Birth of the Living God*. Chicago, IL: University of Chicago Press.

Rizzuto, A.M. (2001). Does God help? What God? Helping whom? The convolutions of divine help. In: *Does God Help? Developmental and Clinical Aspects of Religious Belief*, eds. S. Akhtar & H. Parens, pp. 19–52. Northvale, NJ: Jason Aronson.

Roback, H.B. (2000). Adverse outcomes in group psychotherapy: Risk factors, prevention, and research directions. *The Journal of Psychotherapy Practice and Research* 9(3): 113–122.

Rogers, C.R. (1942). *Counseling and Psychotherapy*. Cambridge, MA: Riverside Press.

Roget, P.M. & Mawson, C.O.S. (1962). *Roget's International Thesaurus* Third Edition. New York: Thomas Y. Crowell Company.

Roland, A. (1988). *In Search of Self in India and Japan: Towards a Cross-Cultural Psychology*. Princeton, NJ: Princeton University Press.

Roland, A. (2011). *Journey to Foreign Selves: Asians and Asian Americans in a Global Era*. New Delhi, India: Oxford University Press.

Rothe, K. (2018). Intimacy: Inner space and relating with others. *Psychoanalysis Today*. Retrieved on February 4, 2018, from www.psychoanalysis.today/en-GB/PT-Articles/Rothe164015/Intimacy-Inner-Space-and-Relating-with-Others.aspx

Rotenberg, M. (1977). "Alienating-individualism" and "reciprocal-individualism": A cross-cultural conceptualization. *Journal of Humanistic Psychology* 17: 3–17.

Rubalcava, L.A., & Waldman, K.M. (2004). Working with intercultural couples: An intersubjective-constructivist perspective. *Progress in Self Psychology* 20: 127–149.

Rubin, L.B. (1986). On men and friendship. *Psychoanalytic Review* 73B: 165–181.

Rubin, T. (1989). Editorial: Intimacy and cultural pressures. *American Journal of Psychoanalysis* 49: 1–4.

Rushkoff, D. (2013). *Present Shock: When Everything Happens*. New York: Penguin.

Russell, G.I. (2015). *Screen Relations: The Limits of Computer-Mediated Psychoanalysis and Psychotherapy*. London: Karnac Books.

Salerno, R. (2014). Changing patterns of intimacy: A review of 'Intimacies: A new world of relational life', ed. by A. Frank, P.T. Clough & S. Seidman. *Psychoanalytic Perspectives* 11(3): 316–320.

Sales, N.J. (2015, September). Tinder and the dawn of the 'Dating Apocalypse'. *Vanity Fair*. Retrieved on February 4, 2018, from www.vanityfair.com/culture/2015/08/tinder-hook-up-culture-end-of-dating

Saul, L.J. (1951). A note on the telephone as a technical aid. *Psychoanalytic Quarterly* 20: 287–290.

Sax, D. (2016). *The Revenge of Analog: Real Things and Why They Matter*. New York, NY: PublicAffairs.

Schaefer, K. (2018). *Text Me When You Get Home: The Evolution and Triumph of Modern Female Friendship*. New York: Dutton.

Schaefer, M.T., & Olson, D.H. (1981). Assessing intimacy: The PAIR inventory. *Journal of Marital and Family Therapy* 1: 47–60.

Schafer, R. (1995). Aloneness in the countertransference. *Psychoanalytic Quarterly* 64: 496–516.

Schaffner, B. (2001). Androgyny in Indian art and culture: Psychoanalytic implications. *Journal of the American Academy of Psychoanalysis* 29(1): 113–125.

Scharff, D.E., & Scharff, J.S. (Eds.) (2014). An overview of psychodynamic couples therapy. In: *Psychoanalytic Couple Therapy: Foundations of Theory and Practice*, pp. 3–24. London: Karnac.

Scharff, J.S. (Ed.) (2013). *Psychoanalysis Online: Mental Health, Teletherapy and Training, Vol. 1*. London: Karnac Books.

Scharff, J.S. (Ed.) (2015). *Psychoanalysis Online 2: Impact of Technology on Development, Training, and Therapy*. London: Karnac Books.

Schimel, J. (1987). On failed intimacy. *Journal of the American Academy of Psychoanalysis and Dynamic Psychiatry* 15: 553–557.

Schopenhauer, A. (1851). *Parerga und Paralipomena, Vol. II*, trans. E.F.J. Payne. Oxford, UK: Clarendon Press, 2000.

Schwaber, E. (2007). The unending struggle to listen. In: *Listening to Others: Developmental and Clinical Aspects of Empathy and Attunement*, ed. S. Akhtar, pp. 17–39. Lanham, MD: Jason Aronson.

Searles, H.F. (1960). *The Non-Human Environment in Normal Development and in Schizophrenia*. New York, NY: International Universities Press.

Senior, J. (2015). *All Joy and No Fun: The Paradox of Modern Parenthood*. New York: Ecco Press.

Shane, E. & Shane, M. (1997). Intimacy, boundaries, and countertransference in the analytic relationship. *Psychoanal Inquiry* 17(1): 69–89.

Sharpe, E.F. (1940). Psycho-physical problems revealed in language: An examination of metaphor. *International Journal of Psychoanalysis* 21: 201–213.

Shengold, L. (1967). The effects of overstimulation: Rat people. *International Journal of Psychoanalysis* 48: 403–415.

Shengold, L. (1971). More about rats and rat people. *International Journal of Psychoanalysis* 52: 277–288.

Shi, Q., & Scharff, D.E. (2011). Cultural factors and projective identification in understanding a Chinese couple. *International Journal of Applied Psychoanalytic Studies* 8(3): 207–217.

Siegel, D.J. (2015). *Brainstorm: The Power and Purpose of the Teenage Brain*. New York: Jeremy P. Tarcher; Penguin.

Slavin, J. (2010). Becoming an individual: Technically subversive thoughts on the role of the analyst's influence. *Psychoanalytic Dialogues* 20: 308–324.

Smith, A. (2012). Part IV: Cell phone attachment and etiquette. *Pew Research Internet Project*. Retrieved on February 4, 2018, from www.pewinternet.org/2012/11/30/part-iv-cell-phone-attachment-and-etiquette/

Smith, A., & Anderson, M. (2016). 5 facts about online dating. *Pew Research*. Retrieved on February 4, 2018, from www.pewresearch.org/fact-tank/2016/02/29/5-facts-about-online-dating/

Smith, P. (1982). Does play matter? Functional and evolutionary aspects of animal and human play. *Behavioral and Brain Sciences* 5(1), 139–155. doi:10.1017/S0140525X0001092X

Solomon, J., & George, C. (2008). The measurement of attachment security and related constructs in infancy and early childhood. In J. Cassidy & P.R. Shaver (Eds.), *Handbook of attachment: Theory, research, and clinical applications*, pp. 383–416. New York, NY, US: Guilford Press.

Spangler, G., & Grossmann, K. (1993). Biobehavioral Organization in Securely and Insecurely Attached Infants. *Child Development* 64: 1439–1450. https://doi.org/10.2307/1131544

Sperling, M. (1952). Animal phobias in a 2-year old child. *Psychoanalytic Study of the Child* 7: 115–125.

Sperling, M. (1971). Spider phobias and spider fantasies: A clinical contribution to the study of symbol and symptom choice. *Journal of the American Psychoanalytic Association* 19: 472–498.

Sroufe, A. L., & Waters, E. (1977). Attachment as an organizational construct. *Child Development* 48: 1184–1199.

Standage, T. (1998). *The Victorian Internet: The Remarkable Story of the Telegraph and the Nineteenth Century's Online Pioneers*. New York, NY: Berkeley Books.

Stein, R. (1998). The enigmatic dimension of sexual experience: The
"otherness" of sexuality and primal seduction. *Psychoanalytic Quarterly* 67: 594–625.

Stern, D.N. (1985). *The Interpersonal World of the Infant*. New York: Basic Books.

Stern, D.N. (1998). *The Interpersonal World of the Infant*, 2nd edition. New York: Basic Books.

Stern, D.N., Sander, L.W., Nahum, J.P., Harrison, A.M., Lyons-Ruth, K., Morgan, A.C., Bruschweiler-Stern, N., & Tronick, E.Z. (1998). Non-interpretive mechanisms in psychoanalytic therapy: The 'something more' than interpretation. *International Journal of Psychoanalysis* 79(5): 903–921.

Stern, S. (2009). The dialectic of empathy and freedom. *International Journal of Psychoanalytic Self Psychology* 4(2): 132–164.

Stolorow, R.D., & Grand, H.T. (1973). A partial analysis of a perversion involving bugs. *International Journal of Psychoanalysis* 54: 349–360.

Stone, L. (2009, November 30). Beyond simple multitasking: Continuous partial attention. *Linda Stone*. Retrieved on February 4, 2018, from https://lindastone.net/2009/11/30/beyond-simple-multi-tasking-continuous-partial-attention/

Stovall-McClough, K.C., & Dozier, M.T. (2016). Attachment states of mind and psychopathology in adulthood. In: *Handbook of Attachment: Theory, Research, and Clinical Applications*, 3rd edition, eds. J. Cassidy & P.R. Shaver, pp. 715–738. New York: Guilford Press.

Strathearn, L. (2011). Maternal neglect: oxytocin, dopamine and the neurobiology of attachment. *Journal of neuroendocrinology*, 23(11), 1054–1065.

Sullivan, H.S. (1953). *The Interpersonal Theory of Psychiatry*. New York, NY: W.W. Norton & Company.

Syasar, Z.S., & Bakhshani, N.M. (2014). The study of sexual function of couples and its relationship with domestic violence. *Journal of Novel Applied Sciences* 3(11): 1308–1311.

Tähkä, V. (1993). *Mind and Its Treatment: A Psychoanalytic Approach*. Madison, CT: International Universities Press.

Tell, C. (2013). Step away from the phone. *The New York Times*, September 22. Retrieved on February 4, 2018, from www.nytimes.com/2013/09/22/fashion/step-away-from-the-phone.html

Thayer, E.C. (1879). *Wired Love: A Romance of Dots and Dashes*. Retrieved on February 4, 2018, from www.gutenberg.org/ebooks/24353

Thompson, M.G. (1998). Manifestations of transference: Love, friendship, rapport. *Contemporary Psychoanalysis* 34(4): 543–561.

Thomson, J.A., & Aukofer, C. (2011). *Why We Believe in God(s)?* Charlottesville, VA: Pitchstone Publishing.

Thorne, B. (1991). The quality of tenderness. In: *Person-Centred Counselling*, pp. 73–81. London: Whurr.

Ting-Toomey, S. (1991). Intimacy expressions in three cultures: France, Japan, and the United States. *International Journal of Intercultural Relations* 15(1): 29–46.

Toffler, A. (1970). *Future Shock*. New York, NY: Bantam Books.

Traub-Werner, D. (1986). The place and value of bestophilia in perversions. *Journal of the American Psychoanalytic Association* 34: 975–992.

Trub, L., & Barbot, B. (2016). The paradox of phone attachment: Development and validation of the Young Adult Attachment to Phone Scale (YAPS). *Computers in Human Behavior* 64: 663–672.

Trub, L., & Barbot, B. (in press). Texting as a means of escape or expression? Development and validation of the Messaging Motivations Questionnaire. *Measurement and Evaluation in Counseling and Development*.

Trub, L., & Starks, T.J. (2017). Textual healing: Proof of concept study examining the impact of a mindfulness intervention on smartphone behavior. *Mindfulness* 8(5): 1225–1235.

Turkle, S. (1995). *Life on the Screen: Identity in the Age of the Internet*. New York, NY: Simon & Schuster.

Turkle, S. (2004). Whither psychoanalysis in computer culture? *Psychoanalytic Psychology* 21(1): 16–30.

Turkle, S. (2011). *Alone Together: Why We Expect More from Technology and Less from Each Other*. New York, NY: Basic Books.

Turkle, S. (2015). *Reclaiming Conversation: The Power of Talk in a Digital Age*. New York, NY: Penguin Press.

Turkle, S., Essig, T., & Russell, G.I. (2017). Afterword: Reclaiming psychoanalysis: Sherry Turkle in conversation with the editors. *Psychoanalytic Perspectives* 14(2): 237–248.

Twenge, J. (2017a). Have smartphones destroyed a generation? *The Atlantic*, September 2017. Retrieved on February 4, 2018, from www.theatlantic.com/magazine/archive/2017/09/has-the-smartphone-destroyed-a-generation/534198/

Twenge, J. (2017b). *iGen: Why Today's Super-Connected Kids Are Growing up Less Rebellious, More Tolerant, Less Happy – and Completely Unprepared for Adulthood*. New York, NY: Simon & Schuster.

Twenge, J.M., & Park, H. (2017). The decline in adult activities among U.S. adolescents, 1976–2016. *Wileyonlinelibrary: Child Development*, September 17. doi:10.1111/cdev.12930

Tyson, P., & Tyson, R. (1999). *Psychoanalytic Theories of Development*. New Haven, CT: Yale University Press.

van Ijzendoorn, M. H. (1995). Adult attachment representations, parental responsiveness, and infant attachment: A meta-analysis on the predictive validity of the Adult Attachment Interview. *Psychological Bulletin* 117(3): 387–403. http://dx.doi.org/10.1037/0033-2909.117.3.387

von Krafft-Ebing, R. (1892). *Psychopathia Sexualis*. New York: Arcade Publishing, 1998.

Walsh, F. (2008). Spirituality, healing and resilience. In: *Re-Visioning Family Therapy: Race, Culture, and Gender in Clinical Practice*, eds. M. McGoldrick & K.V. Hardy. New York: Guilford Press.

Wang, W. (2015). Interracial Marriage: Who is marrying out? *FactTank – Pew Research Center*, June 12. Retrieved on February 25, 2018 from, www.pewresearch.org/fact-tank/2015/06/12/interracial-marriage-who-is-marrying-out/

Weinberg, H. (1989). Clinical aspects of friendliness and friendship. *Contemporary Psychoanalysis* 25: 357–370.

Wheeler, L., Reis, H.T., & Bond, M.H. (1989). Collectivism-individualism in everyday social life: The middle kingdom and the melting pot. *Journal of personality and Social Psychology* 57(1): 79–86.

Wheelis, A. (1994). *The Way Things Are*. Fort Worth, TX: Baskerville Publishers.

Williams, M. (1922). *The Velveteen Rabbit*. New York: Doubleday, Doran & Company.

Wilson, R. (2017). Census: More Americans have college degrees than ever before. *The Hill/The Hill.com*, April 3.

Winch, A. (2013). *Girlfriends: Postfeminist Sisterhood*. London: Palgrave.

Winnicott, D.W. (1953). Transitional objects and transitional phenomena. *International Journal of Psycho-Analysis* 34: 89–97.

Winnicott, D.W. (1958a). The capacity to be alone. In: *The Maturational Process and the Facilitating Environment*, pp. 29–36. London: Karnac Books.

Winnicott, D.W. (1958b). The capacity to be alone. *International Journal of Psychoanalysis* 39: 416–420.

Winnicott, D.W. (1960a). Ego distortion in terms of true and false self. In: *Maturational Processes and the Facilitating Environment*, pp. 140–152. New York, NY: International Universities Press, 1965.

Winnicott, D.W. (1960b). The theory of the parent-infant relationship. *International Journal of Psychoanalysis* 41: 585–595.

Winnicott, D.W. (1963). The development of the capacity for concern. In: *The Maturational Process and the Facilitating Environment*, pp. 29–36. London: Karnac Books.

Winnicott, D.W. (1969). The use of an object. *International Journal Psychoanalysis* 50: 711–716.

Winnicott, D.W. (1971). *Playing and Reality*. London: Tavistock Publications.

Winnicott, D.W. (1984). *Home Is Where We Start from*. New York, NY: W.W. Norton & Company.

Yekta, Z.P., Raisi, F., Ebadi, A., & Shahvari, Z. (2015). Sexual satisfaction concept analysis in Iranian married women: A hybrid model study. *Global Journal of Health Science* 7: 345–353.

Yerushalmi, H. (2013). On the therapist's yearning for intimacy. *Psychoanalytic Quarterly* 82: 671–687.

Young, L.J., & Wang, Z. (2004). The neurobiology of pair bonding. *Nature Neuroscience* 7: 1048–1054.

Zalusky, S. (1998). Telephone analysis: Out of sight but not out of mind. *Journal of the American Psychoanalytic Association* 46(4): 1221–1242.

Zhang, Y., & Van Hook, J. (2009). Marital dissolution among interracial couples. *Journal of Marriage and Family* 71(1): 95–107.

Zeifman, D., & Hazan, C. (2016) Pair bonds as attachments: Mounting evidence in support of bowlby's hypothesis. In: *Handbook of attachment: theory, research, and clinical applications*, eds. J. Cassidy & P.R. Shaver. New York: The Guilford Press.

Zolfaghari, H. (2010). *The Encyclopedia of Persian Proverbs*. Tehran: Moein.

Index